# Praise for *Rewriting Life Scripts:*
## Transformational Recovery For Families of Addicts

"I have found the greatest barrier to recovery is when the family doesn't participate in the programs available to them. This wonderful book tells you why and how the family can help the addict to recover."

Edith Royal, Honoree, Austin Recovery – Edith Royal Campus

"This book will be immensely helpful to family members as they wade into and through a loved one's recovery from drug addiction or alcoholism. It is often presumed that once a loved one enters treatment, all will be fine and return to normal. It doesn't—at least not at first—and having a book like this one that explains, encourages, advises, and offers hope will not only help family members, it will help the addict/alcoholic, as well. Addiction is a family disease and helping the entire family is so important for everyone concerned— *Rewriting Life Scripts* is a must read for all family members of an alcoholic/addict in recovery."

Lisa Frederiksen, author of
*If You Loved Me, You'd Stop! What You Really Need to Know When Your Loved One Drinks Too Much*

"*Rewriting Life Scripts* is a must read for everybody in a family that lives with addiction. A lot has been written about and for people who are addicted. But this book is for the family. And it's good.

Desjardins, Oelklaus, and Watson cover the entire waterfront: understanding the dynamics occurring in families who live with an addicted member, understanding addiction and recovery, and then most important, they give you strategies for dealing with the issues, both your own and that of the addicted member.

Their advice is very straightforward and practical. They actually describe how to let go of guilt and remorse. And their description of the family disease is a very real picture of the kind of reactions family members develop when they live with someone who is addicted. It's true that family members become dysfunctional when they live with addicted people, and don't have the benefit of going through recovery to learn to behave differently. This book should be in the hands of every person who lives with someone in the family or close friendship circle who is addicted. Thanks to the three great women who spent the time to put it together!"

Tony Mandarich, former NFL player,
author of *My Dirty Little Secrets: Steroids, Alcohol, and God*

D1228087

"I found *Rewriting Life Scripts* to be a concise and extremely helpful and informative Handbook and Resource tool, with not only helping the Alcoholic and Addict; but more so for the family that is jeopardized during the pain and wreckage of living in the dysfunction of the Alcoholic and Addict. This book is the perfect bridge for Families who are in desperate need of what they should know, not only what to do in the crisis, but also what is involved in the aftermath of recovery. I learned a lot and have so many friends and families that I will be able to refer this book to. Thanks for writing it!"

Christa Jan Ryan
Author of *Silent Screams from the Hamptons* and *From the Depth of a Woman's Soul*

"While reading *Rewriting Life Scripts,* I easily could visualize myself and my family going through the 'Four Stages of Recovery' mentioned in this book. I agree that family members develop their own set of addictive behaviors while trying so desperately to cope with the addict in the family. Without recognizing it, family members become addicted to: a) how to control situations and events, b) making decisions and excuses, c) intuit when their addicted loved one needs help or a swift kick-in-the-ass, and d) doing whatever is necessary to cope with the stress of the addict's roller coaster ride. *Rewriting Life Scripts* guides family members dealing with an addicted loved one toward hope, common sense, understanding, and restructure. I, personally, would have appreciated reading this insightful book during my own family's struggle with an alcoholic son."

Barbara Sinor, Ph.D.,
Author of *Addiction: What's Really Going On? Inside a Heroin Treatment Program* and *An Inspirational Guide for the Recovering Soul*

"This is without doubt the best book I have read on recovery from addiction. Although the recommendations in the text bear a similarity to my own work with a variety of presenting problems, not only addictions.

I feel honored to have been able to contribute in my role as editor for Loving Healing Press. I can immediately think of half a dozen of my clients who will benefit from reading it.

The book is based on the Twelve Steps made famous by AA. Therefore, it may be particularly useful to those readers who dislike going to meetings and participating in groups. They can get the benefit from here, and perhaps that will give them the courage to face a group."

Bob Rich, Ph.D., Australian counseling psychologist and professional editor.

# Rewriting Life Scripts

## Transformational Recovery
## For Families of Addicts

Liliane Desjardins
Nancy Oelklaus
Irene Watson

Foreword by Douglas Ziedonis, MD, MPH

Cover art designed by Liliane Desjardins, in collaboration with Richa Kinra (colorist).

Library of Congress Cataloging-in-Publication Data

Desjardins, Liliane, 1938-
  Rewriting life scripts : transformational recovery for families of addicts / by Liliane Desjardins, Nancy Oelklaus, Irene Watson.
    p. cm. -- (Life scripts recovery series)
  Includes bibliographical references and index.
  ISBN-13: 978-1-932690-97-2 (trade paper : alk. paper)
  ISBN-10: 1-932690-97-2 (trade paper : alk. paper)
  1. Addicts--Rehabilitation. 2. Addicts--Family relationships. 3. Codependency. I. Oelklaus, Nancy, 1943- II. Watson, Irene, 1946- III. Title.
  HV4998.D47 2009
  362.29'13--dc22
                    2009019030

Distributed by Ingram Book Group (USA/CAN), New Leaf Distributing, Bertram's Books (UK), Agapea (Spain), The Hachette Group (France), Angus & Robertson (Australia).

Published by **Life Scripts Press**, an imprint of
Loving Healing Press
5145 Pontiac Trail
Ann Arbor, MI 48105

Toll free 888-761-6268
info@LHPress.com
www.LHPress.com

# Contents

# Contents

# Acknowledgements

No project of this magnitude springs solely from the named authors. Many people become involved and we would like to formally acknowledge just a few of them:

Bill Wigmore, CEO of Austin Recovery. In conversations with Bill, we realized there was no concise and informative book for families to learn about many aspects of what addiction is, how it affects families, how to cope, and most of all, to know they aren't alone and help is available. Bill had an idea and we filled the need.

Tyler R. Tichelaar, Superior Book Promotions, for his dedicated hours of editing to be sure the content flowed and the reader is able to understand what we are saying.

Victor R. Volkman, Publisher, for believing in our work and making this book possible.

Richa Kinra, for expanding the original cover artwork design by Liliane.

Each of our respective husbands: Gilles Desjardins, Harlan Oelklaus, and Robert Watson. Their support, their candor, and their belief in the work we do enabled us to rise to the need of this book.

# Foreword

Addiction hijacks the brain and the family members of the addict. Alcohol and other drugs hijack the brain's normal functioning and magnify all other problems in the addict's life, including relationships to others in the family. Family members get sucked into the tornado of addiction and can become over-consumed with the addict's behaviors and are fearful of what will happen next. Addiction can ruin the life of parents, spouses, and children who feel they are walking on eggshells and adjusting to the addict's behaviors. Family members seek help and guidance on understanding addiction and what they can do. Ultimately, we realize that we can only change ourselves. However, there is much that can be learned that makes a difference.

Although draining and distracting, the addiction only represents the tip of the iceberg. Underneath the visible addictive behaviors are deeper feelings, thoughts, patterns of behavior, and brain changes that derail the brain from supporting self-awareness and a fulfilling life. Recovery breaks down denial, secrets, and living without awareness. Recovery transforms our old patterns—old "tapes" or "scripts"—that we seem to repeat in our life choices. An important place to start in living our lives is living in the present. Addiction distracts us from awareness, healing, and transformation. Many experiences have led to the current moment and our unique humanness. Transformation and recovery is a journey of self-love and love of others. This book will help many family members increase their awareness and skills for the journey.

For over twenty-five years, I have worked with addicts and always make an effort to include family members. As an Addiction Psychiatrist, I have had the privilege to work in all types of addiction and mental health treatment settings that cared for people from all walks of life—rich and poor, heroin addicts and alcoholics, young and old, men and women—from many cultural backgrounds. From these experiences, I know families go through a common experience with unique aspects. There are core questions and issues. This book addresses the common issues and provides a wonderful guide that I wish I had been able to give out to family members throughout my career. I will in the future.

In addition to my clinical practice, I've had the privilege to work as a faculty member and student with many outstanding clinicians, people in recovery, family members, and clinical researchers and leaders. I've worked at medical schools with world-class addiction research and clinical programs, including UCLA, Yale, University of London, Rutgers University Center for Addiction Studies, and now at UMass and our Center of Excellence in Addiction. Listening to families and addicts has helped me the most in developing my clinical practice skills and in developing the most important clinical research questions that must be pursued. In addition, our UMass research team is uncovering new fundamental discoveries about the impact of alcohol and other drugs on the brain through brain imaging and genetic research, including how these substances change our brains and turn on and modify our genetic code. The blending of the wide range of perspectives in addiction treatment and research has been a personal commitment and journey for me. No one person has all the answers, but there is much out there to help. The understanding of the brain, recovery, and transformation is helpful, but families need practical help and guidance.

About fifteen years ago, I became aware of Liliane (the lead author of this book) and Gilles Desjardins and their Unified Model of Treatment of Addictions. I recognized their incredible wisdom and passion for their work that developed from their many years of clinical and personal experience. The more I learned from them, the more I was impressed with their insights and approach. Their insights have helped my own journey, and I have encouraged students to learn their model to complement other medical and addiction psychiatry approaches. My true admiration of their work comes from seeing them in action with patients and families, in addition to their program's excellent clinical outcomes.

*Rewriting Life Scripts: Transformational Recovery for Families of* Addicts encapsulates the Desjardins' many years of clinical experience into a needed and practical guide for family members in transition. It's a wonderful book that provides both the reality of addiction and its impact on families, but it's also a guide for family members' own journey of recovery. This is a book about hope, forgiveness, and love. Using an engaging style, the book is easy to read and provides practical and effective approaches to supporting family members in recovery. The authors help us learn from stating and answering common questions that family members ask and through the use of helpful exercises that stimulate self-exploration. Families will gain more self-awareness, insight, and skills to improve their relationships and achieve the lives they desire. The "common questions" used in this book are the same that families ask me routinely in my practice, such as "What can we do to help the addict after treatment?"; "How do I let go of guilt?"; "What do you mean it's a family disease?"; "When is it self-love versus selfishness?"; "How are the Twelve Steps helpful?"; "What is a healthy boundary?" "What's the difference between good enabling and bad enabling?"; "How can I try giving up control?"; "What should I look for if I think my loved one is using?"; "How can we communicate better?"

Recovery from addiction is a process, and the book is organized around the four stages all families go through. The first, "Living with Addiction," is a time of increased awareness of the problem; ongoing denial, minimizing, and rationalizing; and powerful feelings of shock, fear, anger, uncertainty, shame, and guilt. Family dynamics change during "wet," "damp," and "dry" substance use periods. Families are awakening to the consequences and living a life consumed by others' behaviors. During the second phase—"Transition to Recovery"—there is a focus on getting help that may include a family intervention. This is a time of setbacks, anger, and ongoing uncertainty, but there are glimmers of hope and frustration with any delays by the addict in seeking help. This is a time when family members may see the need for getting their own help.

In phase three, "Early Stages of Recovery," there is a lot going on. This is a time when the addict's brain is undergoing acute and prolonged detox from substances. It's like the brain is going from being a pickle to a cucumber. There are many symptoms due to brain chemistry changes and adaptations. Just writing this foreword made me realize we really know almost nothing about what happens to family members' brains during this phase, although, through modern science brain imaging, we do know that individuals living under other traumatic contexts do have brain changes due to the trauma and also a healthy brain changes with removal and recovery from the traumatic experiences. I can only assume that family members also undergo change. This is a time when family members are often confused about their roles and even angry that they have a role. There is often an acceptance that they not only have been impacted by the tip of the iceberg (the addiction), but that they have had many other experiences in their earlier life that have shaped who they are and contributed to the current moment. As you read this text, you are in a moment now, one that has developed by an amazing number of events and factors in your past. However, you only have this moment and a limitless range of options for the future.

The fourth phase of the book, "Ongoing Recovery," is one about transformation for the addict and/or the family members. Sometimes either, neither, or both continue on the journey of recovery. The addict will be further working the Twelve Steps and uncovering other possible strengths and problems to address, including mental, psychiatric, spiritual, medical—even other addictions—compulsive behaviors, and tobacco addiction. Family members and addicts see the need for a life plan of wellness and recovery, of transformation, living in the moment, moment to moment, day by day, with new awareness and curiosity, with a zest for life.

The book provides a section of success stories that are very helpful. There is strength and hope found in these profound stories of transformation and healing. Family members will appreciate reading about others' similar experiences and what strategies they used that gave them strength for their recovery. These stories provide a message of hope.

The final section focuses on the family members' recovery and transformation with a guide and review of the Twelve-Step recovery program for family members. Intertwined are helpful examples of common codependent behaviors and roles (such as being a caretaker, people pleaser, workaholic, martyr, perfectionist, tap dancer). Of course, all of us are more complicated than any of these character roles, but these examples provide helpful ways to reflect on oneself and common patterns. The book also has helpful coping skills to increase awareness and realization of what the family can and can't change so that there is increased ability to forgive and apologize while seeking joy, love, trust, laughter, kindness, and hope in all our relationships—with God, self, family, friends, and others. Going beyond just understanding the addict, this section of the book will help family members better understand their own actions and reactions and have a deeper understanding of the drivers of those behaviors. This is not a book about shame and blame. This is a book about meeting families where they are, and gently supporting them to a higher ground—to finding themselves and moving forward.

In summary, this is an important guidebook for family members and has something new to offer them. This book reinforces and augments what therapists, treatment programs, and mutual support Twelve-Step programs provide. Liliane and I have had many conversations about how to help family members and address the family members' need for more information, insight, and strategies during addiction treatment. They commonly have many questions. Change is not easy for any one of us. Addiction grabs the life out of its victims. Life is the journey and the path is not always clear. This book is a wonderful resource and catalyst for change. I am honored to be able to make a very small contribution to this book, and grateful that Liliane and her colleagues are putting this material out for others to use in the context of their recovery and treatment. Family members will gain new insights, learn new skills, and have more hope.

Douglas Ziedonis, MD, MPH
Professor and Chair, Department of Psychiatry
Director, UMass Center of Excellence in Addictions
University of Massachusetts Medical School/UMass Memorial Health Care System

# A Personal Testimony for Rewriting Life Scripts

After seven months of waking up night after night, praying that God would take me away from the pain I was in, I picked up the phone and called Pavillon International and made arrangements to go to their 28-day program, fortunately beginning within a few weeks. For years, I had been hearing from a number of my peers in ministry about how their life had changed through the program. I had also wanted to spend some time getting in touch with my "family of origin issues." Little did I know about what kind of journey I was about to embark on. It was 1995 and as a result of those 28-days, I was changed for life!

What has been most challenging for me during the years since is conveying to my friends and family the astounding impact such a personally-experiential, powerful, and truly unique model Liliane and Gilles Desjardins' have created... challenging to describe because of the transformative personal results known only to each individual. The practical tools, visionary insights, adaptive processes, and unconditionally loving staff and environment , all served to break open the cauterized hearts of many a participant... me included. As a young girl and into my teen years, I was sexually molested by my father. As a married adult woman, I perpetuated the abuse by acting out with numerous affairs (while also fighting a life-long paradoxical battle between codependency and narcissism). Although I had a college degree, a successful career in broadcasting, a license and ordination as a Unity minister, hundreds of friends across the country, a loving husband, and much to look forward to at age 45; I began to believe that there was nothing for me to live for and fell into deep despair and clinical depression.

Within nine days of beginning the program and participating in the Desjardins Model of Treatment, I began to feel *alive* again. Through the work of taking personal inventories, of being quiet and listening to the tall tales I'd been telling myself all these years, of making time for introspection, and opening my heart and mind to "reality checks" and feelings I had never felt before, I began the journey of recovery and healing. Day after day and evening after evening, I experienced shifts in my thinking. I began to recognize the tightly held beliefs and judgments which had been keeping me "safe", yet unavailable to my "life."

Because I became receptive to healing at depth, I experienced the Holy Comforter (or whatever you might call that mysterious or mystical wave of insights and "ah-ha" moments) available and present to me... just for the asking. Whether it was through the teachings of Liliane & Gilles and their staff, the carefully thought out inventories, the stories of others in the program, my personal journaling, etc; these most magical and mystical experiences were happening daily. I recognized that no matter what family environment I grew up in, by hanging on to the old "survival" strategies of yearning to be the "perfect" first child, the "polite" daughter of my southern heritage, a perfectionist and workaholic self... I had actually *lost* my true self. I began the process of *un*covering the truth, in my *re*-covery. It has now been 14 years and I continue to rely on the practices and tools learned from my experience with the Desjardins Model. I now work as a Spiritual Counselor, specializing in addictions, recovery, sexuality, and couples communication... and am pursuing my Doctorate in Pastoral Counseling. In these years since working the Model, I have rarely felt that I was not here for a reason... a purpose. And I have continued to grow in ways beyond my wildest imaginings. *This* is the truth that indeed sets one *free*!

As you read the pages ahead, dive totally and completely into the material, the practices, the questions, and the journaling. You can rest assured you are stepping into sacred territory and you will not be hurt, judged, nor abandoned. You will be embraced in compassionate and loving care. Within each chapter, there are practical and provocative tools offering concrete answers and definable steps for knowing *how* to live in a recovering family. You will be reaping the rewards of many who have gone before you, successfully using this proven family recovery model; through your Divine purpose while discovering new meaning in your life. And as you become totally open and receptive to the journey ahead, may you also experience more and more *moments* of freedom. This will bring more Aliveness to your life and the lives of those you love. Get ready to be changed at depth... through wisdom, grace, and unconditional love. You will never want to go back!

Carolyn R. Craft,

Broadcaster, Visionary Producer/Developer, and Business Executive and Advisor

# Introduction: Families in Recovery

Having a loved one in recovery for an addiction can be difficult for family members who have been so preoccupied with the addict's behavior that they have forgotten to take care of their own needs. Family members may feel lost, not knowing how to replace the time and worry spent over the addict, or how to continue to help an addict who has begun recovery.

This book has been written to guide the recovering addict's family through an understanding of what the addict is experiencing during recovery and to help the family members learn to let go of the pain from the past, undergoing their own recovery from the chaos and trauma caused by the addict's behavior. During the loved one's addiction, family members may have tried to help the addict or control the addict's behavior. They may have denied the addict has a problem. They may have spent so much time trying to take care of the addict that they have not taken the time to care for their own needs. Now is that time.

Where does recovery for the family begin? Some recovery centers have family programs, but so many questions remain unanswered. Recovery is sometimes a difficult and painful process of deep-seated and fundamental change that is not easy and rarely is smooth for families. Without knowledge about what to do or expect, including knowing what is normal and necessary, change can be disruptive and traumatic; without a clear path for recovery, the family members may cause more harm to themselves and perhaps to the addict. This book lays out the process of recovery for the family members themselves.

Recovering family members must go through four stages:

- **Practicing addict** has substance abuse (living with addict prior to recovery)
- **Transition** of addict into recovery (addict goes into a recovery center)
- **Early stages of recovery** (learning, abstinence, change; family members are confused about their roles)
- **Ongoing recovery** (addict continues abstinence; family is guided by values of recovery)

In the early stages, the family's environment and family dynamics can get out of control. Each family member must enter into a personal recovery, shifting individual attention away from the addict and the unhealthy family system that was created by the addiction. All family members must focus attention on themselves, learning new tools to deal with the behaviors formerly used to cope with having an addict in the family. The family's reactions, attempts to control the addict, or denial of the addiction served to protect the family at times; at other times, these behaviors only fueled further destruction of the family unit. Now, new tools must be acquired. New responses and coping behaviors must be learned so that family members can communicate with each other. Most importantly, each family member needs to experience a personal recovery—freedom from the pain and craziness that resulted from the addict's behavior.

Outside support networks, such as Twelve-Step programs and therapy, are usually the only ways family members can substitute the unhealthy system with a healthy environment. In the end, we realize that recovery for families has a positive outcome; it creates a foundation for in-depth change however difficult the journey may seem.

With understanding, family members can turn their relationships within the family into positive outcomes without threatening the recovery process of the addict, their own stability, or that of other family members. Understanding, growth, and hope can take place when family members are open and receptive to education and support; and most of, all willing to "work" on themselves, on their own fears and manifestations. As families come together and as individual family members progress in their recoveries, the environment becomes safer and a new healthy family develops. How and when this transformation occurs depends on the individual family. It is our hope that the following pages will help you develop a healthy family.

# Part I:
# Understanding Addiction
# and the Recovery Process

<table>
<tr><td>

# 1

</td><td>

# Low Bottom vs.
# High Bottom Phenomenon

</td></tr>
</table>

Between 1935 and 1938, Alcoholics Anonymous (AA) was founded by and for low bottom alcoholics, that is people who had lost everything due to their alcoholism and were on skid row or close to it.

After *The Big Book of Alcoholics Anonymous* was published in 1938, alcoholism became less of a taboo and moral issue. Over the years, due to publicity and the emergence of rehabilitation centers, it became less and less of a taboo.

In 1954, thanks to Marty Mann, the U.S. Congress recognized alcoholism as a treatable disease. At that time, other phenomena entered the stage including: prescription drugs, marijuana, and soft drugs. "Pure alcoholics" became cross addicts, switching from one substance to the other, using a little of everything to keep the constant buzz, without outer evidence of heavy intoxication. Of course, some even crossed the line into heavy and illegal drugs.

Due to this fact, society's perception of who is an alcoholic stayed the same as in 1935: a low bottom, skid row drunk. Today, such people represent only 4% of the total addicted population. Thus, a lot of people qualify as addicts, but due to their social and economic status, they are not diagnosed as such.

Some treatment facilities have adjusted their programs to this new phenomenon of high bottom addicts and, as a result, are starting to treat behavioral addictions as well as substance addictions. Behavioral addictions are called *Process Addictions*.

A few typical Process Addictions are:
- Workaholism
- Food addiction—eating disorders
- Sex addiction, cybersex, pornography etc.
- Relationship addiction
- Romance addiction
- Gambling
- Smoking (nicotine)

Process Addictions get their name from the fact that they are a process. The difference from abusing a substance is that in that situation the addict quits using the substance, works a program, and his/her disease gets arrested and treated. Process addiction is different: people continue working, eating, having sex etc. Therefore, they must learn how to manage the process of that addiction and learn a different behavioral response to stress, pain, and life.

We rarely see an addict with just one addiction. Most addicts know how to switch from one to the other. Dr. Patrick Carnes and his colleagues, Robert Murray and Louis Charpentier, in "Addiction Interaction Disorder" (*Handbook of Addictive Disorders: A Practical Guide to Diagnosis and Treatment*), have very well identified the interaction between different addictions and the reasons for it.

It is important to know and understand the addict's behavior in early recovery, as many addicts will give up their main identified addictions only to switch to others. Example: the heroin addict gives up heroin and picks up methadone. The alcoholic gives up alcohol and switches to workaholism or sex addiction. The addict's behavioral patterns are still going to be dysfunctional and if not addressed, can lead back into using substances.

## Understanding the Family Process

It is well known in the addiction treatment community that addictions affect those close to the using person in many ways. The pain, embarrassment, and sense of loss may be overwhelming for family members. This mindset often continues when the addict receives treatment because there is a different set of variables that families must overcome: what to expect when the addict returns home and how to respond to the addict's behaviors.

Unlike the recovering addict, the addict's family members may have limited knowledge and understanding about the recovery process. Very few treatment facilities have adequate training for families other than a cursory overview of what the addict went through in recovery. The importance of having the family's questions answered is often compromised, thereby not preparing the family to understand the addict's behaviors or how to give support.

In the Desjardins Unified Model of Treatment of Addictions, substance addictions and process addictions represent 15% of the problem. They are the medicators the addict uses to medicate the other 85% of the disease. That other 85% is the cause of the addiction, the pain the addict tried to cover up with the addictive substances in an attempt to make the pain go away. The 85% of the disease is a state of mind, composed of specific psychological tendencies, emotional patterns, imprints, and the inflated or diseased ego. Today, science knows that alcoholics and drug addicts have a genetic predisposition to substances. It is handed down generationally although it can skip a generation or two.

The addict who quits using alcohol, drugs, or any process addiction medicator (nicotine, food, gambling, sex, relationships, or work), faces the full impact of the above stated psychological tendencies and emotional patterns and responses. The addict's feelings are no longer medicated and numbed with substances and medicators, without having yet mastered a healthy new way to respond to life.

In treatment, the addict learns how to deal with and process these emotional states without medicators. The addict usually completes treatment with good intentions. Promises are voiced to commit to the recovery process. In most cases, positive changes can be seen immediately.

However, a return into daily circumstances often triggers old patterns of behavior that were used to cope with the pain, thus creating a great need for ongoing recovery. To family members, it might look like the person is relapsing...and they are, not necessarily into substances but rather into old behavior patterns. The addict may not respond or behave in ways that reflect being in recovery, or may behave in ways the family sees as unproductive. For family members, this new reality may feel overwhelming, especially when their efforts of encouragement and support seem inadequate.

Below are the psychological tendencies of people in recovery. If these tendencies are not observed and used as warning signs, they may push a recovering addict into a relapse of old behavior patterns, including the return to addictive substances.

## Psychological Tendencies of the Addict

- **Low Tolerance to Circumstances:** This tendency is the most common. It is the incapacity to endure any inconvenience or suffering for a long time. The person cannot accept any sentiment or circumstance that is unfavorable.

- **Grandiose Appearance:** It is the universe turning around "Me, Myself, and I." The person puts on a protective shield to hide feelings of inadequacy and devaluation. Although the person projects nice images of himself, his personal and intimate convictions of his worth are low; his value is diminished; and he suffers from an inferiority complex. The person does not feel adequate but dares not show it.

- **Anxiety:** All people experience some anxiety, but this person suffers from it in an exaggerated way. He is subject to all sorts of apprehension and fear. Usually he is not certain of himself, or the reason for his anxiety.

- **Perfectionism:** The person affixes for himself objectives so high that it is impossible to attain them. This results in feelings of defeat and guilt, causing suffering he cannot endure and for which he needs relief or escape.

- **Isolation:** Due to an exaggerated need to protect his intimacy, the person begins to retreat from others and society; he develops the behavior of a solitary person. This makes it difficult to make permanent and sincere friends.

- **Illusionary Thoughts:** The person becomes a master in the art of arranging things so they seem reasonable. He may twist the truth, withhold information to make himself look good, or invent stories to cover up the truth. He tends to tell the truth as he sees it.

- **Hypersensitivity:** The person has a tendency to exaggerate in all his interpersonal relationships especially when things are not favorable. He is easily hurt and he nourishes hurt feelings for long periods so that they become the basis of his resentments.

- **Impulsiveness:** "I want what I want, when I want it, now." Often the person is proud to be impulsive, and he considers this a good quality. In reality, his impulsiveness only brings more tension.

- **Defiance:** This is the result of unbearable inner conflicts and anxieties. The person feels rejected by others, whether or this is true. Since he feels he cannot properly belong to the group, in order to defend himself, he defies people who want to get close and help.

- **Dependence:** The dependence on others becomes exaggerated. It is caused by the person's immaturity and is usually followed by feelings of hostility toward the source of his dependence.

## Addiction Process

Addiction and Recovery form a process, both for the addict and the family. Here we will illustrate this process.

1. **The addict starts occasional relief usage (drinking or drugs).**
   Family members might even enjoy this period as the addict may be more relaxed and pleasant under the influence.

2. **The addict's usage becomes more frequent, even regular.**
   Family members feel neglected and/or abandoned and excluded from the addict's life. Doubts and resentments build and family members start complaining.

3. **The addict contrives excuses, alibis, and justifications.**
   Family members start the pattern of *control* in search of truth.

4.  **The addict's level of tolerance to substances increases; memory blackouts start. The ability for rational thinking decreases and the urgency for the first drink or drug increases.**

    Family's level of powerlessness increases, due to lack of understanding of the disease process. The crazy-making continues shifting powerlessness into anger and resentments. This is confusing as the family loves and hates the addict at the same time. In many cases, the family will start manifesting illnesses: stomach aches, migraines, backaches etc.

5.  **The addict's level of responsibility and family involvement decreases and guilt and shame level increases, causing the addict to be oversensitive to any criticism, expectations, and demands by the family members.**

    Frustration level, control level, and anger level by family members increase while trust, hope, and respect for the addict decrease. The cycle of loneliness is established.

6.  **The addict loses the ability to stop using when others do, covering that loss with grandiose and aggressive behaviors coupled with persistent remorse. The addict multiplies efforts to control the usage and fails. The addict makes promises and resolutions and fails.**

    The family's trust is shattered; yet, codependence keeps the family members on the merry-go-round of denial, minimization, shame, blame, and enabling the addict to keep behaving badly without consequences.

7.  **At this stage of the progression of the disease, the addict isolates from the family,** tries geographical escapes, and experiences loss of other interests. Work and money problems start. The addict neglects his/her appearance as well as proper nutrition. This will be followed by the loss of power of choice, loss of rational thinking, as well as responsible decision-making. Unreasonable resentments, blame, and feelings of paranoia are now a daily state of the addict's mind and their purpose is to hide the guilt, shame, and deep sense of repeated failure. Moral deterioration follows.

    The family has joined the addict at this stage. The addict is obsessed with getting the next drink/drug and the family is obsessed with fixing, changing, or saving the addict. The family members become co-addicts. Sometimes family members will seek outside help; however, the unspoken rule of not revealing family secrets prevents many from doing so. The families who seek outside help often manage a successful intervention and the addict enters treatment. However, some will go through divorce and bankruptcies.

8. **The addict's level of tolerance to substances has diminished,** which will cause the onset of lengthy intoxications, multiplying impaired thinking periods. The addict will seek the company of chronic users and will start a period of indefinable fears. These will be followed by the inability to initiate actions as the addict is totally obsessed with using. Being intoxicated is the only escape from the inner turmoil of self-hatred.

   The family is exhausted, overwhelmed with responsibilities, making excuses, internalizing the sense of failure that the addict feels. The addict is failing in promises and control of the substances; family members are failing in their efforts to change the addict.

At this phase, the addict has exhausted all the alibis and will experience vague spiritual desires. This is the point where some addicts will admit defeat and have an honest desire for help; however, many will end in prison, bankruptcy, or death.

For the fortunate ones who choose recovery, a new cycle begins.

## Recovery Treatments

Before we can successfully look at the recovery process and the sequence of improvements, it is important to remember that results and quality of recovery vary according to treatment philosophy and program in place. There are a variety of approaches to treatment of addictions:

- Biopsychosocial model of treatment of addictions
- Pharmacopsychosocial model of treatment
- Holistic model of treatment
- Twelve-Step based model of treatment
- Integrated models of treatment, combining different therapies and modalities with the Twelve-Step approach
- Christian-based programs

Addictions are complex and so are the treatments. It is important for the family members to understand the model of treatment their loved one has received; it will save the family a lot of misunderstandings.

Whether the addict has undergone treatment or simply joined a Twelve-Step Group, there are common and recognizable improvements that will follow as the Recovery Process starts.

## Recovery Process

1.  **The addict enters recovery via a treatment facility or Twelve-Step Program.**

    At this point, the addict has stopped using and has discovered that addictions are a treatable illness that can be arrested. The prerequisite to sustained sobriety and recovery will be abstinence and change of lifestyle. It is also the period of withdrawal and learning how to face life, reality, and stress without the habitual medicators. The entire biological system has been affected and medical evaluation is crucial. Another important factor at this stage: the addict meets recovering addicts whose lives are happy, healthy, and functional. The addict is encouraged to examine his/her life and is assisted in the personal stocktaking. This is the period of hope and release of the first layers of guilt. The right thinking begins.

    The family members at this point are usually confused. On one hand, they are relieved and hopeful: the insanity produced by intoxication has stopped. On the other hand, they are left with all the unanswered questions, doubts and fears: is this going to last? Who is this new person? When is he/she going to be "normal," responsible, and present to family? The list of expectations is long, and the memory of broken promises is not erased.

2.  **The addict is involved in the recovery process: the tremors subside, the cravings diminish or are eliminated, and memory gets restored.**
    Energy level and concentration ability greatly improve with proper nutrition and regular sleep. Family members are delighted with the visible physical and mental improvements, and they assume that the emotional improvements are matching the rest. They assume that the addict is now "normal" and therefore responsible and capable of putting the family's needs first. Some family members still wrestle with old resentments and the fact that the attention was centered on the addict before and still is.

3.  **Feeling much better and healthier, at the third month mark, many addicts feel they have won the battle and they have the addiction "under control."**
    Their attendance at the Twelve-Step meetings or group therapy changes; they are back in charge and dealing with life's stress and circumstances in the old way. The "stinking thinking" is back. They are stuck and denying it. They are on a "dry drunk," exhibiting neuropsychological impairment and neurotoxicity.

    The last person they will listen to for advice is a family member. Actually, at this point, they become defensive and start avoiding, blaming, justifying their behavior, and using alibis. A good sponsor in a Twelve-Step group or a caring peer or therapist will be able to reach them and pull them back into the program.

Needless to say, the family members are confused, angry, fearful, rejected. Their main question is, "Are we back to square one? When is this crazy-making going to stop?" Many spouses at this point start considering divorce or some other drastic measure. Many shut down emotionally and sexually, creating additional stress in the relationship and being stuck between guilt and anger. The need for family members to enter their own recovery process rapidly increases.

4. **If the addict rejoins the program, a new period of growth will follow.**

   The addict has realized that doing it alone is not working. Usually, this is the point where the addict examines his/her spiritual needs, values, and beliefs. A new level of honesty and humility follows. The addict starts appreciating the possibilities of a new way of life. The addict's fears of the unknown future diminish. Sobriety is getting stabilized and so are the addict's emotions. This is the beginning of the return of self-esteem.

   The family's trust starts to rise. If the family members have joined a recovering community and started working on their anger, resentments, fears, and control issues, they are starting (in a parallel way with the addict) to get better. For many, *control* has become a permanent state of mind. To be told they must surrender is incomprehensible, the premise being, "If I don't do it, who will?"

   Between the sixth and ninth months of sobriety, the addict's need to escape has diminished and his/her thinking is more realistic. The addict starts to adjust to the family's needs. Many try to re-establish their positions of authority in the family, which in many cases is met with the family's resistance. Many try at this point to resolve the financial crisis and/or stress caused by years of active addiction. Some even have to face legal or work issues.

   This is a new possible crisis point. Once again the stress is mounting, and the medicators are no longer there. Depending on the seriousness of issues, the crisis is building, the tunnel vision returns, plans begin to fail, and self-confidence is very shaky. Due to lack of coping and communication skills, problems with family, work, finances etc. multiply and the addict feels victimized.

   Some addicts become immobilized: daydreaming; engaging in wishful thinking; feelings of futility; grandiose thoughts of career, relationship, or even geographical change. Daily tasks are being procrastinated and recovery neglected.

   At this point, Addiction Interaction Syndrome kicks in. Some addicts will use process addiction medicators such as food, gambling, workaholism, or sexual acting out to numb the inner turmoil. Some addicts will escape into sexual fantasies and masturbation, while others will medicate with cybersex and pornography, causing even more damage to the precarious intimacy of their relationships.

All these medicators can bring temporary relief. However, if not confronted with his/her behavior by a sponsor, a caring peer, or therapist, and brought back to the program, the addict will continue on this self-defeating path.

5. **The addict is confused and overreacts with anger, blame, and feeling misunderstood. Depression returns, bringing with it old patterns: poor nutritional choices, irregular sleep, loss of desire and structure, and periods of profound sadness.**

For some, loss of control will follow: the addict rejects help, dwells in self-pity and lies, starts thinking of using again, is overwhelmed with loneliness, frustration, and anger. The addict is isolated and has pulled away from all support. The options at this point are: go back to using, go crazy, or commit suicide.

Through this turbulent period, the family is on the same ride as the addict. The family goes through an endless range of emotions: fears, doubts, anger, jealousy, insecurity, inadequacy, as well as self-rejection and guilt. For the family, the addicts' return to old, destructive, or dysfunctional behavior patterns is frightening and devastating. Having not gone through recovery, they may feel helpless, not knowing what to do to help the addict. They struggle with many questions: what should we do when we see behaviors contrary to what we believe are correct for a recovering addict? First of all, the family has to answer the question: Are we feeling responsible for not doing enough or not supporting the recovering addict with these struggles?

In most cases, the answer to that question is "Yes." One of the reasons is that family members do not know what to do when things appear to change for the worse. They agonize over how or why addiction happened to their family. They seek assurance that the addict will recover. They hope to understand that they did not cause it—they cannot cure it and they cannot control it. Someone told them there were no guarantees.

At this point, it is important for family members to know that there is something they *can* do—and that is to take action to help themselves, one day at a time.

The first action for the family at this point is to get an understanding of the process of addiction and recovery and to join a recovery program or therapy.

Many families choose to do that; yet others initiate divorce and/or custody battles as they feel they cannot cope with the situation any longer.

6.  **For most addicts, at this turning point, an intervention and firm confrontation by a sponsor, a peer, or therapist will produce a "wake-up call" that brings them back into the program of recovery.**

    That is when the real recovery work kicks in. The addict faces his/her illusionary thought pattern and starts a spiritual recovery process.

    New interests are developed, and a new circle of stable friends is acquired. The addict's perceptions of a "Sponsor" role changes. The addict is becoming receptive and teachable. The sponsor or therapist is no longer perceived as an authority to be resisted, but rather as a life coach. This is the period of new values and ideals.

    The addict has accepted the fact that recovery must come first, which means that the principles of recovery must be practiced in every area of his/her life. The addict makes amends and is repairing the damages of the past by a profound change in his or her behavior and attitude.

    Family and friends appreciate the addict's new attitudes and efforts and usually at this point, the family has joined the addict in recovery. Now, the true family rehabilitation begins. New tools are being acquired: how to identify feelings and process them. The importance of being in the now moment is understood and becomes a way of not projecting the past into the future.

7.  **The addict has gained a new ability to face facts and unfavorable circumstances with courage. Forgiveness and self-forgiveness are slowly becoming a natural way of being and the addict now operates from values anchored in recovery principles.**

    At this point, the addict and the family are starting to experience an increase in emotional manageability and stability.

    This is another pivotal time in recovery. It happens around the first year of sobriety. It is the beginning of emotional maturity. Some addicts will take the first steps toward economic stability while others will take steps toward responsible fiscal stewardship. The addict is regaining the confidence, respect, and trust of employers or of his employees and society. By now, the addict has discovered the value of service work and sharing. The habitual selfishness, egotism, and self-righteousness are being replaced with compassion, empathy, generosity, and a desire to grow. Needless to say that the addict's self-esteem increases and is experiencing joy and contentment in sobriety.

8.  **The addict's perceptions have shifted. From seeing recovery as a punishment, boring and restrictive, the addict is discovering a new creativity, a deeper meaning to life. The addict values his or her newfound ability to connect emotionally with other addicts as well as with family.**

    Family members are experiencing relief, joy, hope, and trust. However, in some cases, the spouse may be jealous of and threatened by all these new friendships the addict has. The same feelings can apply to the sponsor.

    New resentments will be built f the spouse feels left out of decisions that concern the family, yet the addict resolves them with his or her sponsor only.

    The family is glad the addict has help, yet feels left out. It is an important phase for family members as their perceptions, expectations, and needs are challenged and need to be worked through.

    This is the point where family therapy and couples' work are important. Partners in recovery will spell happy relationship and fulfilling sobriety and recovery for all.

9.  **The addict's level of tolerance for stress is now greatly increased. The addict easily recognizes his or her rationalizations, character defects, and ego behaviors. The addict has gained the ability to de-dramatize and not take self so seriously.**

    The family's perfectionism, expectations, and control have been replaced by a new ability to surrender, accept, and trust. Past wounds have had time to heal. The boulevard of broken dreams is no more the sad street on which they live. New hope, new goals, new values are in place, and the family is gaining a new sense of self-respect. They do not feel as outcasts any longer.

    The addict and the family feel enlightened at this point. An interesting way of life has opened up and the road of recovery now leads to discoveries, spiritual growth, and maturity. Integrity, commitment, responsibility, accountability, connectedness, intimacy etc. are no more just words; rather, they are a new way of being.

> "Sobriety isn't the goal of recovery;
> it's the *prerequisite* for recovery."
> —Jack Boland

| **2** | # Frequently Asked Questions From Family Members |
|---|---|

## What can I do to help them after treatment?

In most cases, recovery is a whole new experience, not only for the addict, but also for the family and friends. When someone seeks out treatment, it generally means the person has had a breakdown in communication in his relationships; the best thing to do is to re-open the lines of communication. This can be done by:

- Asking the newly recovering addict how we can support him or her
- Establishing ground rules about the consequences if unacceptable behaviors occur
- Paying attention to our own feelings and expressing them
- Being honest
- Refraining from blaming by using "I" statements
- Establishing our own support system through sponsors (CODA, Al-Anon)
- Seeking outside help for ourselves
- Doing nothing (sometimes leaving him or her alone may be the best option)
- Looking for the changes and praising him or her for them, no matter how small they are.

## Why is *this* person the addict?

Parents especially ask this question. They want to understand how they can have one child who is fine, often even an over-achiever, while another child becomes an addict. How is this possible when the children come from the same family with the same parents?

When we really think about it, no two children are ever born into the *same* family. When the second child is born, the parents are a different age, it is a different year, and there is an older sibling. Family circumstances change and affect children in different ways. And then there is the issue of genetics.

The same question could be asked in families of blondes who birth a brunette or families of high achievers who birth a child with a learning disability. And the list could go on and on.

This is not a useful question to ask or try to answer. Instead, we encourage using our brainpower to achieve acceptance. A starting point is to say the Serenity Prayer every time this question comes up.

*God, grant me the serenity*

*To accept the things I cannot change,*

*Courage to change the things I can,*

*And wisdom to know the difference.*

The only thing we can change is ourselves; our attitude. What we choose to think about. How we choose to feel. Remember: what we resist, persists. So try acceptance.

And remember: this addiction is not about you.

## What does the Serenity Prayer mean?

*Serenity* is a peaceful state of mind. When we have serenity, we are at our best. That is, we do our clearest thinking and remain calm from an inner sense that, regardless of the circumstances around us, within us all is well.

*God, grant me the serenity*

*To accept the things I cannot change*

Serenity comes from letting go of the attempt to control things that are beyond our ability to change. We cannot control how other people drive or how much alcohol other people consume or how anyone behaves. Much of our turmoil comes from trying to change things that are beyond our power to change.

Try this: Make a list of things you are powerless over. For example, other people being on time, the service at a restaurant, choices made by other people, the color your neighbor chooses to paint his house, the nose ring worn by the teller at the bank, the weather. You cannot control these things. Quit trying and you'll feel better. Keep adding to this list for a week, and then read back through it at the end of the week. Realize how much energy you have expended trying to control things you are powerless over. This is energy that you could be using to create the life you truly want to live.

Then there's the next line:

*courage to change the things I can*

That means us. What we do have power over and can change is ourselves. We ask for the courage to make the internal changes needed to live in a peaceful state of mind. This courage comes with awareness of when we are being judgmental and critical of other people. The serenity prayer calls us to detach from what other people are doing and set a higher standard for ourselves. This takes courage.

The root word of *courage* means *heart,* which is where we find:

*wisdom to know the difference*

We stop using our heads to try to figure things out and solve the problems. Instead, we get in touch with our own hearts, start listening to them, and begin to make the changes WE need to make. This wisdom to know the difference dawns slowly over time. Many people find it helpful to read something daily that opens their abilities to discern between what we can and cannot control. The daily reader entitled *Courage to Change* is an excellent source. Other sources are listed in the bibliography.

## Can someone give me a definition of codependency that makes sense?

The glossary for the Desjardins Unified Model of Treatment of Addictions defines codependency as "a learned behavior expressed by dependencies on people to the point of diminishing one's identity: a state by which a person's sense of value and self-love are based on other people's opinions of him/her, allowing himself/herself to be made or broken by them."

At www.coda.org is a very helpful checklist of characteristics of codependents. In general, we who are codependent can say how everyone else is feeling, but not how we are feeling; in other words, we "absorb" others' feelings and do not speak up on our own behalf. We feel we are not worthy, and we strive to please other people instead of ourselves.

Another way of looking at it is that the alcoholic/addict is dependent on alcohol or drugs; the codependent in relationship with the addict *depends* on the addict for self-worth. We become co-addicts who "lose" ourselves. It's not uncommon for codependent spouses, as the addiction progresses, to narrow our world. We stop going out with friends. We abandon things we enjoy doing. We don't invite people over. We allow the addict's behavior and habits to control how we live our lives and how we react to situations.

Author Lisa Frederiksen in her book entitled *If You Loved Me, You'd Stop!* asserts:

Just as there is a series of chemical reactions taking place in the brain of an alcoholic or abusive drinker, so too is there a compulsive-like process occurring in the codependent's brain…The repeated surges of adrenaline required to keep you safe in a dysfunctional home—always on high alert in order to uphold the family rules—cause your brain to eventually REACT *without* THINKING to hundreds of situations…This constant high alert level of reactivity eventually becomes a chronic state of hyper-vigilance. This causes the codependent's brain to become comfortable with a heightened level of adrenaline (and other related neurotransmitters and hormones) and angst. That comfort level then becomes 'grooved,' if you will...and allows a codependent to experience the unacceptable as acceptable. (p. 49-50)

Gilles Desjardins, co-founder of the Desjardins Unified Model of Treatment of Addictions, puts it this way, "What the codependent is powerless over is their *reaction* to the alcoholic or addict."

(Complete details on codependency are in Chapter 12.)

## What are the "stages of change"?

As often heard in Al-Anon meetings, the stages of change are: awareness, acceptance, action. From listening to families of alcoholics and addicts in meetings and from talking with our own sponsor, we become aware of how we are contributing to dysfunction and enabling the addiction. This awareness is not a one-time event; it is recursive in that we do it again and again as we become increasingly aware of the dynamic of addiction and our part in it.

This brings us to the second stage—acceptance. We fully accept that we are powerless to change the past. And we are powerless over addiction. We stop trying, in the words of the Serenity Prayer, to "change the things we cannot change."

Then we find "the courage to change the things we can." This is the action step. And what can we change? We can change our own feelings. We can change the choices we make. We can change how we live our own lives, regardless of anyone else's choices and behaviors. We can do what is authentic for us, living one day at a time, forgiving ourselves and every other person.

Family recovery is not a course of study that one completes and then moves on. It is an ongoing process of ever-deepening one's capacity to live a happy life, free from attachments to other people's choices and behavior. Sustaining this ongoing process includes going to Al-Anon meetings, talking regularly with a sponsor, reading the daily readings, working the steps, and performing service work to support the group.

Often we go to Al-Anon and start to feel better. So we stop going. Then, a year or so later, we come back, writhing in pain. This pain is unnecessary. All we have to do is keep going back and not stop. The Al-Anon program of family recovery is about living a happy life, free from emotional turmoil. It's about having a peaceful state of mind, no matter what. It works as long as we keep going back and practicing the principles of the program.

## How do we let go of our guilt?

This question is asking for some action, so we're going to describe some actions that are guaranteed to release guilt.

One of the first slogans learned in Al-Anon is, "You didn't cause it. You can't cure it. And you can't control it." Say this slogan over and over. Every time we feel guilt, we say to ourselves, "I didn't cause it. I can't cure it. And I can't control it." When we keep saying these words to ourselves, we begin to detach. We write them. We post them on our bathroom mirrors or refrigerator doors—or both. We do whatever it takes to remember.

We write out what we're feeling guilty about. We put a lot of emotion into the writing. We feel all of our feelings. Then we put these sheets of paper through a shredder and listen closely to the grinding sound of the shredder as the pages go through. From that moment on, each time we feel guilt trying to come back into our conscious awareness, we remember the sound of the shredder and say to ourselves, "It's gone. I shredded it." If we do not have a shredder, we burn the pages. When the memory tries to come back, we smell the smoke and remember that it is gone.

We find a place outdoors with lots of rocks and no other people. We gather a pile of rocks and think about what we feel guilty about. We pick up one rock at a time, with one guilty feeling in mind. We press the rock hard with our fingers, imagining we are moving the energy of guilt from our bodies into that stone. Then, when we are ready, we throw the rock/guilt as far away as we can. We release the guilty feeling with the rock. We deeply feel the relief and remember it when guilt tries to creep back into our consciousness (and it will try).

Processes like these are effective because they involve the emotional and physical as well as the mental. The mistake most of us make is that we try to "figure it out," which is a mental process. Thus, we keep going round and round in our minds, like a hamster on a wheel. This does not work.

Being authentic is a journey of acknowledging that we are powerful spiritual beings and co-creators with God. When we remember this truth, we move away from endless negative mind chatter and move directly into our hearts. This space is where our true essence, our knowing, resides—where we align our hearts with God, and ask God to help us see ourselves as God sees us, without any judgment or expectations.

When we live authentically, we act on the guidance we receive; we refuse to let our ego or personality question that guidance. Trusting our guidance is essential. We must always remember that what we need to know and do will be revealed to us in perfect timing.

"The key to change...is to let go of fear."
—Roseanne Cash

| 3 | **Understanding Addictions And Recovery** |
|---|---|

We paid for our son to undergo 90 days of treatment. Only two-and-a-half weeks into the process, he left the treatment center, got drunk, and created a ruckus. Long story short, the treatment center threw him out. Now he's on the streets, with temperatures below freezing. Here's what I don't understand: regardless of whether or not he thinks he has a drug and alcohol problem, he has the opportunity for three meals a day and a warm bed for 90 days. All he has to do is cooperate. Why won't he do it?

## Addiction = Non-Growth

Addiction is a way of staying stuck, repeating the same patterns that do not work like a robot, over and over and over again, and each time thinking the addiction, that next drink, that next high, is going to wipe away the pain. It never does. Taking a phrase from the Big Book, many AA members describe their disease as "cunning, baffling, and powerful." Here's a story from someone in recovery:

Once I heard of a program for children of alcoholics/addicts sponsored by a treatment center. Part of the program included a puppet show depicting the addict in two forms. One, the person he/she truly is: a kind, thoughtful, loving person—the sober one—the person who brings gifts, and encourages. The person you trust to do the right thing. Behind that person, however, was a puppet that depicted an unruly, disrespectful, angry person who looked just like mom or dad and acted badly. A person who made you afraid and confused—someone who could never be trusted. And with this parent, you never knew which puppet you would get.

This puppet show was a way of helping children distinguish between the person and the addiction. It was a way of saying their parent was really two people—their true, authentic self and their unruly, unreasonable, baffling self attached to their addiction.

## Addiction = Attachment

- When we are attached to something or someone, we have forgotten who we are.

- We feel we cannot be whole without this something.

- We experience pain and suffering whenever our attachment threatens to leave us.

- Attachment is the cause of suffering.

## What is Recovery?

The following is a true life story:

My husband and I are both in recovery: he, for alcoholism; me, for codependency, workaholism, and compulsive overeating. I'll keep the focus on myself and say that my dependence on what other people thought, my perfectionism, my need to be right, and my need to be in control caused me a great deal of emotional pain. In other words, I was ill at ease in this world. I didn't feel that I fit. I didn't trust people—not anyone. I did not realize how my mind had been shaped by growing up in an alcoholic home. I kept trying to prove that I was good enough. Mostly, I did this through my career, in which I was very successful. I was the one who made things happen. I knew how to "call the shots," and I was *attached* to the results. Now I realize that I could have been as successful—maybe even more so—had I been working and living out of my authentic self and not my ego.

What I've learned in recovery is to let go. I've learned I am enough. I don't have to be right. I can be wrong and still be loved. It's okay to have my faults. I'm working on them, but I'm no longer striving for perfection. I can laugh at myself. I can see what I'm doing and say to myself, "Well, there you go again!"

What I love most about recovery is admitting my powerlessness. It's a paradox, and I've found it to be true that there is great power in powerlessness.

Today, I don't feel stressed. I am at peace. When someone tells me a scary story or expresses intense anger, I say to myself, "I'm powerless over that." I don't have to fix it or get involved. I can have compassion and say what I truly need to say without fear. For me, to be able to truthfully say this has taken years.

Today, when I wake up in the middle of the night with something on my mind, I say to myself, "I'm powerless" and keep repeating it until I drop off to sleep, which doesn't take long at all. Most of the time, I am free of fear and anger. I have forgiven myself and everyone else—for everything.

Recovery isn't a check-off list; it's first and foremost developing a treasured relationship with a Higher Power. Once that relationship is established, living in recovery is exquisite, continuously deepening one's relationship with and delight in God.

I've learned that God has a sense of humor—that miracles are all around me, every day—that God can and will do for me what my ego cannot do. I've learned that I'm so much more than what I do or how much money I have or what people think about me. I've learned I am enough, and I have enough.

The lifelong process of recovery begins with letting go—surrender—powerlessness—non-attachment.

## Recovery = Non-Attachment

- Non-attachment does not mean non-caring. It means non-needing, non-obsessing.

- Non-attachment removes emotional investment so that one can truly see clearly and therefore care appropriately for the other's sake.

- Recovery is transformation.

- Transformation is transmutation of energy.

- When our energy is not wasted and/or blocked by the diseased ego, then our positive qualities just naturally flow and start expressing.

- Fear is transmuted into courage.

- Self-pity and blame shift into a desire to take personal responsibility for our lives.

- Powerlessness is transmuted into passion.

- Self-preoccupation shifts into an aspiration to serve and give.

- Mood swings balance into a state of serenity.

- Fragmented knowledge is transmuted into holistic truth.

Addiction Is About Past Or Future.

Recovery Is About *Now*.

# 4 | The Dysfunctional Highly-Stressed Family

To better understand our family roles and dynamics—why we behave like we do—we need to look back at our own upbringing. Growing up in a dysfunctional family, we may have experienced trauma and pain, anxiety or confusion from our parents' actions, words, and attitudes. Because of the trauma we experienced, we were probably different from other children, possibly missing parts of our childhood when we were forced into uncommon roles within the family. For some, the pain of the past has led us to substance abuse. For some, we began to repeat behaviors, we learned in childhood, with our own children or spouses. We may feel internal anxiety, anger, or rage without knowing why we feel as we do.

We must not blame ourselves. We must accept that as children we were innocent; our lives were directed by the forces within our family—a family we had no control over. Now, as adults, we are coming to terms with the past; we are adult survivors.

The following exercise will give you insight into what characteristics influence your behavior now.

## Assessment of Family Dysfunctions

Check off the characteristics that were true in your family while growing up. For each check, place to whom it applied.

- ☐ Death of parent or family member:

- ☐ Chronic illness:

- ☐ Divorce:

- ☐ Alcoholism:

- ☐ Drug abuse:

- ☐ Chemical dependency:

- ☐ Grandparents with alcoholism:

- ☐ Gambling:

- ☐ Food addiction (anorexia, bulimia, obesity):

- ☐ Sex addiction:

- ☐ Sexual abuse, incest:

- ☐ Sexual abuse, other:

- ☐ Abuse—Physical:

- ☐ Abuse—Emotional:

- ☐ Abuse—Mental:

- ☐ Abuse—Spiritual:

- ☐ Violence:

- ☐ Workaholism (money, success, prestige-oriented, business building):

- ☐ Emotionally absent or emotionally overbearing parents:

## Core Issues in Dysfunctional Families

- Abandonment
- Low self-esteem
- Abuse Issues: sexual, physical, emotional, religious, financial
- Neglect
- Difficulty or inability to trust
- Lack of honesty and being real
- Feelings are suppressed, repressed, depressed, or angrily expressed
- Dependence fostering neediness
- Difficulty or inability to grieve losses
- Black-and-white thinking and behaving
- High tolerance for inappropriate behavior
- Over-responsibility for others
- Being out of touch with and neglecting our needs
- Avoidance of or difficulty resolving conflict
- Difficulty or inability to face confrontation and unpleasant situations
- Difficulty giving and receiving praise
- Difficulty giving and receiving love
- Difficulty establishing intimacy at all levels, not just sexual
- Secretiveness and hidden agendas
- Instability and irresponsibility

## Roles within Dysfunctional Families

A dysfunctional family is one where the relationships between the husband and wife or the parents and children are strained and abnormal. This often happens when one of the family members has a problem that impacts every member of the family; each member then feels compelled to adapt atypical roles within the family structure as a survival mechanism. Dysfunctional family systems produce delusions, compulsivity, frozen feelings, low self-worth, and/or medical complications.

For example, the wife covers for her problem husband, such as telling his boss he is sick when he has a hangover, so he can maintain employment. She may become so obsessive about her husband's abnormal behavior that she loses perspective on her own life, often termed as codependency. (We will cover this issue later in this book). Sharon Wegscheider, in her book *Another Chance*, referred to this family role as an Enabler. The Enabler protects and takes care of the problem spouse, called the Dependent. The Dependent is not allowed to experience the negative consequences of his actions. Deep inside, the Enabler feels angry and resentful of the burdens placed upon her by her Dependent husband's unhealthy and irresponsible behavior, and she feels powerless to do anything other than cover up for him. She feels she must cover for him if the family is to survive. She takes on the responsibility and often does not have her own needs met, which may lead to stress-related illness. Furthermore, the Enabler's behavior ultimately prevents the Dependent from correcting himself and stopping the downward spiral of addiction.

The children also assume roles within the family to make up for the absence of parenting. These roles within the family are defined as the Hero, the Rebel, the Lost Child, and the Mascot.

## Family Dynamics: The Disease

Dysfunctional family systems produce:
- Delusions
- Compulsive behavior
- Frozen and silenced feelings
- Low self-worth
- Medical complications

Dysfunctional family systems are composed of six major roles:

| | |
|---|---|
| **The Dependent:** | The Addict |
| **The Codependent/Enabler:** | The Spouse |
| **The Hero:** | The Oldest Child |
| **The Rebel:** | The Second Child |
| **The Lost Child:** | The Third Child |
| **The Mascot:** | The Fourth Child |

The following chart indicates the inner state of mind of the person playing each of these roles and how that manifests in the person's behavior.

---

### The Dependent/Addict

**Inner State of Mind**

- Mental:  Preoccupation. Obsessed with maintaining supply of substances. Guarded. Defensive. Suspicious.
- Will:  Powerless
- Physical:  Tense and stressed (sometimes neglected; no rest)
- Social:  Alone, isolated, or ultra-social (is into extremes)
- Emotional:  Afraid—Hostile—Lonely
- Spiritual:  Guilt—Shame

**Outer Behavior (What they look like to an observer)**

- Self-centered and self-absorbed
- Egotistical
- Aggressive
- Self-righteous
- Grandiose
- Selfish
- Denies feelings and reality
- Charming, manipulative
- Dictatorial, controlling

## The Spouse: Codependent Enabler

**Inner State of Mind**

- Mental:  Preoccupation with saving and protecting the addict. Peace at all cost. Controlling. Overwhelmed.
- Will:  Responsible for everyone.
- Physical:  Tired, exhausted, digestive problems, migraines.
- Emotional:  Angry, afraid, guilty, jealous.
- Spiritual:  Codependent relationship with God or angry at God.

**Outer Behavior (What they look like to an observer)**

- Compliant—Submissive
- Passive-aggressive
- Controlling—Critical
- Perfectionist
- Justifying—Excusing
- Self-rejecting
- Over-responsible
- A martyr

## The Hero: The Family Caretaker

**Inner State**

Fearful, insecure
Inadequate
Unimportant
Guilty, ashamed
People-pleaser
Oversensitive
Sad, grieving
Feels like a failure
Secretive (keeps family secrets)

**Outer Behavior**

Compliant, obedient
Over-achiever, competitive
Over-responsible
Perfectionist
Caretaker
Lonely
High suicide rate
Isolated and enmeshed with the
    enabler

**Characteristics**

A fixer
Needs attention and approval
Suppresses feelings and negativity
People-pleaser
Perfectionist
Oversensitive
Self-centered
Silenced feelings
Self-righteous
Intolerant and demanding

**Strengths**

Generous
Very dedicated
Strong in adversity
Very resourceful
Reliable and dependable
Devoted and caring
Has a great sense of justice
Deep inner-life and great values
Forgiving of self and others
Compassionate & understanding

**Solution:** Let the hero know that he/she is okay as is;
no need to be a super hero.

## The Rebel (Compliant/Defiant): Problem Child

**Inner State**

Angry

Fearful, insecure

Hurt and rejected

Jealous, envious

Lonely

Resentful

Judgmental

Willful

False pride

**Outer Behavior**

Quiet, sullen

Withdrawn

Defiant and rebellious

Critical, rejecting

Strong peer group

Overpowering, controlling

Manipulative

First candidate for chemical use

**Characteristics**

Egotistical

Savior

Troubleshooter

Speaks up/blames

Arrogant, defiant

Victim (dwells in self-pity)

Family's scapegoat

Rejects others

Resentful and angry

Needs to belong

**Strengths**

Loyal and devoted

Sees beyond the obvious

Securing

Honest and blunt

Bright and perceptive

Intuitive

Risk taker

Great leader

Faithful protector

**Solution:** The rebel needs and wants acceptance and a sense of belonging. Let him/her know that he/she is wanted and belongs.

## The Lost Child: The Forgotten Child

**Inner State**
Confused
Fearful, insecure
Hurt, sad, and lonely
Shy
Worries a lot, is overly agreeable
Has frozen feelings (due to neglect)
Feels victimized and neglected

**Outer Behavior**
Quiet
Solitary
Withdrawn and isolated
Inadequate
Difficulty relating & communicating
Looks for rewards
Escapes into books and pets

**Characteristics**
His/her existence is ignored
The OK child—has no needs
Needs to do things alone
Indecisive
Procrastinates or delegates
Rationalizes and analyzes
Intolerant
Does not want to lead
Has a deep reflective inner life
Loves to teach
Is a private person
Does not like responsibilities; needs
    An escape route

**Strengths**
Good listener
Present to others
Great student/observer
Soothing, tender
Devoted
Supportive
Forgiving and respectful
Great team player
Grateful and generous
Perseverant
Good boundaries
Great planner/punctual

**Solution: Keep drawing them out of their isolation.**

## The Mascot: Family Pet (The Clown)

**Inner State**
Guilt
Shame
Inadequacy
Fearful and insecure
Loneliness
Has difficulty belonging
Is funny

Worries a lot
Needs to be heard and
    secured

**Outer Behavior**
Hyperactive
Clown; center of attention
Immature and fragile
Feels unimportant
Manipulative
Avoids situations
Diffuses family tension by acting out
    and using humor
Is impatient and demanding
Ridicules and rejects others with
    sarcasm and by being cynical

**Characteristics**
Selfish and immature
Impulsive
Obsessive and compulsive
Dwells in self-pity and drama
Exhibits inappropriate humor
Lacks a sense of timing
Provides relief in the family
    dynamic

**Strengths**
Great sense of humor
Playful
Enthusiastic
Very creative
Is candid,  childlike inquisitiveness
Is a great entertainer for children
Great communicator

Solution:  Needs to be taken seriously.
Acknowledge their being, their strengths, and their skills.

If there is an only child, he or she may take on parts of all these roles, acting out simultaneously or alternately. This often leads to overpowering confusion and devastating pain as a result.

The longer a dysfunctional role goes on, the more inflexible it becomes. In the end, family members become addicted to their own roles, considering them as essential to the family dynamics and acting them out with the same compassion, compulsion, and delusion as the Dependent plays his or her role as the addict. Family dynamics then truly become a family disease.

In case there is a fifth child, he or she will assume the role of second hero. The roles repeat themselves with each additional child. The younger children are greatly influenced by their older siblings and are more estranged from the parents. As the older siblings leave home, many times the younger ones will be cast into a double role, their own and the one the departed sibling had. Needless to say, this just adds to the family dysfunction.

# Questions About
# The Disease

## What do you mean it's a *family* disease?

The following story, as told by an adult child of an alcoholic, reflects how an alcoholic parent can affect the entire family—including the children long after they have become adults themselves.

My father was an alcoholic. Although my parents were divorced, Dad was a tornado in our lives when I was growing up. He would whirl in, be violent (once he even tried to kick down the front door), and whirl out. He didn't contribute financially to child support, so Mother sewed, and Dad's parents helped us out from time to time with a car and clothing.

In my sophomore year of high school, I discovered alcohol, and my family role soon became that of scapegoat. I lost my college scholarship because of my drinking. Then I lost my marriage. After my divorce, I had lots of relationships, like a revolving door. The last man I was involved with, I made my god. When we broke up, I thought my world had come to an end. I hit bottom.

Until then, Mother had been my enabler. She bailed me out of jail, took care of the cars I wrecked, and fixed everything when I overdrew my bank account. But the night I called to tell her I was going to commit suicide was her last straw. She said, "If you need to kill yourself, then so be it."

The next day, I went into treatment for the disease of alcoholism. A doctor I saw there told me that if I didn't want to be crazy anymore, I must stop drinking.

The treatment center suggested I tell Mom about Al-Anon, and she went for about six weeks and then stopped. My relationship with Mother was rocky. She had no boundaries. She would draw a line, but when I crossed it, there would be threats, but no consequences.

Mother supported my recovery by babysitting my son while I went to meetings, but it's been a hard road for the two of us.

Eventually, I went back to school and finished my law degree. After I graduated, Mother, my son, and I celebrated by going to Disneyworld. We had a great time and enjoyed being together.

When it's just Mom and me, we get along great. But when you add my two sisters into the mix, it's awful. No matter how hard I try, I'm still the scapegoat, and anything that goes wrong has to be my fault.

My baby sister is the hero of our family. She never does anything wrong—or so my mother thinks. My middle sister is the peacekeeper, but she'll choose my baby sister over me every time. *Why?* Because I'm the scapegoat.

I know my mother and sisters talk about me and my business behind my back. Recently, when I confronted my baby sister about this, Mom called me a bitch. I have decided I'm not going to be the scapegoat anymore. A family reunion is coming up. The reason for the reunion is that my great-aunt is dying; only no one will admit it. Mom isn't being honest about her real reason for holding the reunion. I know two things: (1) I've told my great-aunt how much she means to me, so our relationship doesn't need this event. (2) When the whole family is together, it's toxic for me. I don't feel free to be who I truly am; my family makes me the scapegoat and the angry one. I'm outnumbered—the only one in recovery. So I have decided not to go.

I'm happy. I have a great life. I don't want what they have. Something has to put an end to this pattern. I'll start with my decision not to go.

In the story above, only one member of the family is in recovery—the addict. But the imprint of the raging father is still very much present. The family system is not healed. In a healthy family system, a mother does not call her daughter a bitch. There are no favorites. Healthy families are loving, kind, respectful, truthful, and forgiving. We don't try to control each other's behavior, and we discipline ourselves to stay in a loving state of mind, no matter what.

In families where addiction is present, the stress of unpredictable, unacceptable behavior puts everyone on the edge. We feel as if we are "walking on eggshells." This is why we call it a "family disease." The family system is ill at ease. The family is dysfunctional.

According to the Desjardins Unified Model of Treatment of Addictions, there are core issues for individual members of dysfunctional families and also core needs for the family itself.

## Core Issues for Dysfunctional Family Members:

- Abandonment
- Low self-esteem

- Abuse issues: sexual, physical, emotional, religious, financial
- Difficulty or inability to trust
- Dishonesty and not being real
- Feelings are suppressed, repressed, depressed, or angrily expressed
- Dependence fostering neediness
- Difficulty or inability to grieve losses
- Black-and-white thinking and behaving
- High tolerance for inappropriate behavior
- Over-responsibility for others
- Being out of touch with our needs and neglecting our needs
- Avoidance or difficulty resolving conflict
- Difficulty or inability to face confrontation and unpleasant situations
- Difficulty giving and receiving praise
- Difficulty giving and receiving love
- Secretiveness and hidden agendas
- Instability and irresponsibility

## Needs of Dysfunctional Families

- Usually the addict's needs polarize the family. Family members are out of touch with their needs and the addict's wants set the tone.
- Part of the family disease is that needs become suppressed while the addict's wants govern, creating a deep sense of resentment and loneliness within the family.
- Suppressed, ignored needs create a deep sense of victimhood and alienation.
- Our authentic self is in touch with what we need, but codependency, fear, and insecurity prevent us from stating our needs.
- We cannot have healthy boundaries unless we know what we need and we assume responsibility for our needs and stop expecting someone else to fulfill them.
- Wants can be congruent with our needs or conflicting.

The following chart was developed as part of the Desjardins Unified Model of Treatment of Addictions to name our needs in spiritual, mental, emotional, physical, sexual, and financial categories of life. The chart illustrates statements we make—to ourselves, as inner talk, or to others—when our wants conflict with our needs. The column to the far right is what we say to ourselves and believe in our hearts when our wants are congruent with our needs.

| Category | NEED | WANTS Conflicting | WANTS Congruent |
|---|---|---|---|
| Spiritual | • To be connected to my God. <br> • To feel sustained. <br> • To feel God's presence. <br> • To feel surrendered. | I want to party. <br> I don't want to give up Diseased Ego. <br> I want to do it my way. <br> I want control. | I want to face and process Ego. <br> I want my quiet time. <br> I want a sponsor. <br> I want a support group. <br> I want to give up my addiction. |
| Mental | • Order <br> • Discipline <br> • Clarity <br> • Consistency <br> • Awake-alert <br> • Organization <br> • Stimulation | I want to party. <br> I want to hang out. <br> I want to do it but… later. <br> Procrastination. <br> Let me watch some more TV. <br> Let me fix it for you. <br> Let me help you. <br> Let me take care of you. <br> I can do it better. | I will clean my room, my desk, my files. <br> I will get up earlier every day. <br> I'll watch what I say. <br> I'll make a sincere effort to be present. <br> I set goals, make a plan of action, and follow through. <br> I allow others to be themselves, to make their mistakes, or have their successes. |
| Emotional | • Love <br> • Support <br> • Peace <br> • Affection <br> • Tenderness <br> • Encouragement <br> • Nurturing | I keep on blaming, complaining, criticizing, gossiping, being insensitive and disrespectful of others. <br> Self-centered. <br> Focused on me. | I give hugs and kisses to others. <br> I want to be generous, present, supportive, affectionate, respectful. <br> I am teachable. <br> I'll sponsor someone. <br> I'll be a facilitator at my support group. <br> I'll be present to my family. |

| Category | NEED | WANTS Conflicting | WANTS Congruent |
|---|---|---|---|
| **Sexual** | • Playfulness<br>• Creativity<br>• Spontaneity<br>• Variety<br>• Feel connected<br>• Tenderness<br>• Permanency<br>• Commitment | I want to stay in a power play.<br>I want control.<br>I want to protect myself.<br>I want to have sex, wherever and with whomever I want. | I want to be present, involved, vulnerable, and close.<br>I want to let go of pretenses and guards.<br>I want to be honest in expressing needs, preferences.<br>I want to be playful and contribute a sense of humor.<br>I want to create a safe environment for both of us.<br>I want to be committed. |
| **Financial** | • Autonomous<br>• Prosperous<br>• Generous<br>• Stability<br>• Security<br>• Integrity<br>• Tithe | I want to spend what I want, when I want.<br>I want to live without a budget.<br>I want to be stingy and miserly and take from others.<br>I want to get it any way I can. | I want to be wise and responsible.<br>I want to be free of debts and generous.<br>I want to tithe. |

In their unified method of treatment, the Desjardins get even more specific about getting clear on needs in the area of marriage. In marriage, they affirm, we have a need to belong, and we also need manageability. Since marriage is a spiritual relationship involving three entities—God, ourselves, and our spouse, the Desjardins developed the following chart to help people get clear on which needs belong to each of these three entities—so that we avoid confusion about our true needs and where they reside.

## NEED: <u>TO BELONG</u>                    AREA: <u>MARRIAGE</u>

| God | Me | Spouse |
| --- | --- | --- |
| I NEED: <br><br>• To feel God as the center of my marriage. <br>• To feel I am on my own path and not trapped in a codependent relationship. <br>• To feel loved and supported by God. <br>• ME as an expression of God in that marriage. <br>• An exciting, vibrant, passionate, and loving connection. <br>• To feel fulfilled so I can give. | I NEED: <br><br>• To be present. <br>• To be committed and consistent. <br>• To be loving. <br>• To be patient, humble, honest, and real. <br>• To be true to me. <br>• Dignity. <br>• To be giving. <br>• To be responsible. <br>• Maturity. <br>• Integrity. <br>• To be caring and affectionate. <br>• Good deeds. <br>• Generosity. <br>• Gratitude. <br>• Acceptance. <br>• Understanding. <br>• To quit playing games. <br>• Sexual connections, e.g.: I need to be sexually present, connected, and playful vs. expecting, and demanding vs. I act as a kid and expect my spouse to treat me as a lover. <br>• I need to be responsible emotionally and financially. | I NEED: <br><br>• Affection. <br>• Tenderness. <br>• Support. <br>• Trust. <br>• Respect. <br>• Honesty |

## NEED: **FOR MANAGEABILITY**          AREA: **MARRIAGE**

| God | Me | Spouse |
| --- | --- | --- |
| I NEED: | I NEED: | I NEED: |
| • A new set of values.<br>• To restore my moral code and boundaries to sanity.<br>• Enthusiasm.<br>• Strength.<br>• Faith.<br>• Love.<br>• God's support and guidance on an hourly basis.<br>• A tough, loving sponsor who will be my role model in relationships.<br>• A "custom-made" sponsor I can give to and feel useful. | • Sobriety.<br>• Abstinence.<br>• Freedom from sex addiction.<br>• Freedom from $$$ addiction.<br>• Freedom from control addiction.<br>• Freedom from suffering addiction.<br>• Willingness.<br>• Humility.<br>• Teachability.<br>• To be open, receptive, honest.<br>• To be caring, interested, involved.<br>• To quit codependent behavior: caretaking, people pleasing, playing martyr, workaholic, perfectionist, tap dancer.<br>• Clear, specific, honest communication.<br>• To learn how to live alone.<br>• Autonomy.<br>• To take my responsibilities at all levels.<br>• The capacity to humbly admit my wrongs and learn.<br>• To grow up. | • An autonomous spouse.<br>• A recovering spouse.<br>• A God-centered and sober spouse.<br>• Honesty and humility.<br>• Understanding.<br>• Integrity.<br>• A responsible spouse free of codependent behavior — one who does not act as caretaker by fixing and saving me—by taking over my responsibilities.<br>• One who does not bail me out in the name of love.<br>• One who does not manipulate the kids.<br>• A lover.<br>• A partner, etc. |

## What does "selfish disease" mean?

An addiction does not consider the needs of any person. It demands to be fed, no matter whom it hurts. It is entirely self-centered. It can convince a drunken person to get behind the wheel of a car with her children in the back seat. It seeks its own pleasure, with no regard even for the wellbeing of loved ones. Thus, it is a "selfish disease," pleasing itself, immune to the hurt it is causing.

- Within the family system, others may also be exhibiting selfishness. Here are the forms it takes, as defined in the Desjardins Unified Model of Treatment of Addictions:

- Selfishness—Preoccupation with self; wanting things MY WAY.

- Self-centeredness—Having or recognizing the self as the center of all things: ME—ME—ME; it's all about ME.

- Self-righteousness—Feeling superior, feeling justified, being egotistical.

It's very easy for the family of an addict to fall into self-righteousness. After all, the addict is out of control and clearly wrong. So others must be right—right? Wrong! In a family with addiction, everyone exhibits selfishness (How dare they interrupt my life?), self-centeredness (If he's drinking, I must have done something wrong. How can I make this right?), and self-righteousness (I'm the sane one, and I know what's good for other people).

## What is the difference between self-love and selfishness?

Acts of self-love are those that feed the soul and strengthen the heart. They are life-giving, health-promoting acts. Some examples might be long walks, nutritious eating, naps, exercise, saying what we truly need to say, meditating, reading literature that lifts our hearts, making lists of what we are grateful for, building a sound financial base, being a good citizen, having lunch with a good friend, writing about and collecting pictures of what a good life looks like, learning tools for how to create a good life for ourselves. Sometimes self-love requires working with a counselor or coach to help us get clear on what we truly want.

If we create a good life for ourselves, others around us benefit as well.

Selfishness, on the other hand, does not come from the heart; it comes from the ego. It says, "I want what I want, and I don't care what you think about it or how it makes you feel." It is self-indulgent and does not regard the deep desires of the heart.

## How can someone be addicted to prescription drugs? (a doctor gave them, right?)

The following story illustrates how even people who have recovered from substance abuse are liable to relapse. Prescription drugs are often a culprit in putting the recovering addict back into an addiction situation. The following story is one woman's experience:

My sister was the only family I had. She lived about three hours away and was a very secretive person. In 1984, she called me out of the blue and told me she had drunk so much that she thought she was going to die. Until that moment, I had no idea she had a drinking problem. I didn't know what to do.

On the advice of a friend, I checked her into rehab. As for myself, I didn't get involved. I didn't go to family week. I didn't go to Al-Anon. When she got out of rehab, she started going to AA. For twenty-one years she was sober. She went to meetings, showed up on time, and did everything her AA friends suggested.

I take pain pills for fibromyalgia. My sister, on the other hand, was very active and healthy—until about two years ago, when she started hurting all over. I don't know what her diagnosis was, but she started taking a lot of pills. I took her to an excellent hospital, but no one could ever find out what her problem was. Her AA friends told her she would have to start over with sobriety. I thought they were awful for telling her she had to start over after she had been sober for twenty-one years.

She checked into another treatment facility. This time, I went to family week, and by now I had been a member of Al-Anon for about three years. I was starting to get it that there was alcoholism in my family. I remembered an uncle who was a funny drunk. We used to laugh at him and make jokes when he landed in jail. Ironically, he outlived everyone and quit drinking at about the age of seventy-eight.

At the conclusion of my sister's second treatment, after twenty-one years in AA, the center recommended she go to aftercare, but instead she went back home and continued to use. Her tolerance was so high that the pills just didn't work to relieve her pain. After she died, I learned she had even made a trip to Mexico to buy drugs. I knew she was very depressed, but I didn't know what to do about it. Her death was ruled a suicide.

For a couple of years, I was very angry at AA and stopped going to Al-Anon. After all, a doctor prescribed those pain pills. What can you do when you are in pain? I got so angry at her AA friends for coming down on her for not working the program with her drug addiction.

But now I understand that alcoholism is a progressive disease. That means, even if you are sober, the disease continues to progress so if you eventually use drugs or alcohol again, your tolerance is so high that it takes a mega-dose for you to feel any effect at all. It's as if you never quit drinking. I now realize that when my sister started taking pain pills, she substituted them for alcohol and was actually feeding her addiction. Although I don't like how her AA friends dealt with my sister, their fears were well grounded.

My advice is that when dealing with an alcoholic with a medical problem that seems to require pain medication, find a doctor who has specialized training in the disease of alcoholism first and can prescribe a course of treatment that does not interfere with recovery.

## What does tolerance to drugs or alcohol mean?

The more people continue to drink or take drugs, the greater the tolerance they build up, causing them to need to take increasingly larger doses to attain the "high" they seek. The following story reflects how an addict builds up that tolerance. The following is an excerpt from one woman's experiences:

> My husband is a very large man. When we first started dating, I noticed he could drink a lot and not appear to be drunk. One night at dinner, I asked him how many glasses of wine he could drink without being drunk, and he said, "Six."
>
> I was so naïve that I believed he could drink a lot because of his size. I did not realize that six glasses of wine is excessive, even for a big man.
>
> Later, I learned that over the forty or so years, he had been binge drinking; he had developed a high tolerance for alcohol. I also learned that even after six glasses of wine over dinner, after I went to bed, he drank even more. It took an awful lot of alcohol for him to "get drunk."

## What does progression of the disease mean and why is it important?

Alcoholism and drug addiction is a *progressive* disease. That means, even if we are sober, the disease continues to progress so that if we eventually use drugs or alcohol again, our tolerance is so high that it takes a mega-dose for us to feel any effect at all. It's as if we'd never quit drinking.

> "It is not because the truth is too difficult to see that we make mistakes... we make mistakes because the easiest and most comfortable course for us is to seek insight where it accords with our emotions—especially selfish ones."
>
> —Alexander Solzhenitsyn, Nobel Laureate

| **6** | # Questions About<br># The Program of Recovery |
|---|---|

## Why should I get help when I'm not the one who's addicted?

Words from some Al-Anon prologues say, "Changed attitudes can aid recovery." Since addiction indicates an illness in the family system, then our job is to heal the illness within us. We do our part, and we do it for two reasons:

- It will help us.
- It improves the chances that our loved one will be successful with recovery.

Here's a story of how getting help by a person helped her daughter's recovery.

My daughter's addiction was my first awareness that alcohol was a problem in our family. I remember my husband on the phone, with a beer in his hand, finding a treatment center for her. At the time, I couldn't see that my husband had a problem, too.

When I was growing up, my dad drank a lot. He would wake me up at midnight just to talk. I was embarrassed by his drinking and his behavior. My husband, on the other hand, didn't drink like my dad—and he was very successful in his career, so he didn't fit the stereotype in my head of what an alcoholic looked like.

After my daughter entered treatment, we went for three days of family treatment. For the first time, I felt I really belonged in that group. But our family still didn't fully face the issue of my husband's alcoholism. I just focused on my daughter and became so interested in recovery that I got trained in family counseling. In my work with families, I found that most families aren't interested in recovery for themselves. Their attitude is, "Not interested. Just fix the kid."

What brought me into Al-Anon was my daughter. She was sober a few years, but then she started "going out," as they say. Then her sister went with her to a Halloween party and afterward reported to me that she was drinking again. From my training as a family therapist, I knew not to confront her. I gave her to God and let her walk her path.

She had several failed relationships. By then, she had graduated from college and just wasn't doing well. She came home, and when she arrived at our home after seventeen straight hours of driving, she was so thin—like a little wounded bird. I had no idea the problem was alcohol; I thought she was cured! And I never asked the question.

On her own, she decided to go to AA, where her fellow alcoholics gave her counsel and advice. After the meeting, one of the women told her, "If you're living in your parents' home, you have to tell them what's going on."

When she did, I decided that her path is her own, and I needed to go to Al-Anon. I began to realize what craziness I was dealing with in my home. I started to become aware of how controlling my husband was. Before Al-Anon, I used to confront him and threaten to leave. But he made all the money, and I was intimidated. He used to say things like, "If you leave, how will you pay for the kids' college?" In Al-Anon, I learned that I had to stop making threats and let the program walk me through the difficult times.

Some devastating things happened in our family. Al-Anon helped me to focus on one thing at a time and to know that I don't have to have all the answers. I just do what I need to take care of me, and let tomorrow take care of itself.

Eventually, my husband went through a treatment program, but he is not in recovery. He's not drinking, but he doesn't have the peace of the program. We're in marriage counseling, and I pray that he comes into the full joy of recovery.

If I didn't have the peace of the Al-Anon program, I'd be a divorced, angry, scared person. But now I know that every problem doesn't have to be solved today.

## What is a Twelve-Step meeting?

When someone we love struggles with drugs or alcohol, panic and desperation are often our first companions. We ask, "What can I say or do to make her stop?" We look for a switch that turns on the light and banishes the darkness. But addiction is complex and intertwined. A single word or action won't change it.

Bill W., one of the founders of Alcoholics Anonymous, discovered after much searching that the solution lay in working what is now known as the 12-Steps of Alcoholics Anonymous, in sharing stories with other alcoholics in recovery, and in service to other alcoholics. When she saw how well this process worked for him, his wife Lois formed Al-Anon for families and friends of alcoholics. Al-Anon adopted the 12-Steps, which are now the backbone not only for AA and Al-Anon, but for other recovery programs, as well, like Overeaters Anonymous and Codependents Anonymous.

The Twelve Steps are the "figure eight" of recovery. If you want to "skate" your way to a happy life, the Twelve Steps are basic. Without them, there is risk of becoming embittered and rigid, not being able to enjoy the full range of emotions. Within the Twelve Steps is the process for forgiveness and recovery of self-respect and appreciation for others.

In Twelve-Step meetings, people share their experiences, strength, and hope related to addiction and relationships with addicts and alcoholics. The purpose of regularly attending Twelve-Step meetings is to hear success stories, find solutions to common problems, and gain encouragement from being with people who have found "contentment and even happiness" through practicing the principles of Twelve-Step programs, "whether the alcoholic is still drinking or not."

Some meetings have open discussions, and we are free to say anything we need to say. Other meetings are more focused and disciplined on working the Twelve Steps, and attendees are asked to stick with the step that is designated for that meeting.

A Twelve-Step meeting lasts for only one hour. A volunteer leader opens the meeting with reading the preamble and announcing the topic. Then the leader either calls on people to speak or they do so voluntarily. Sometimes there are long pauses in the meetings. In this time, we can simply close our eyes and say the Serenity Prayer silently until someone speaks again. The silence can be very calming. We never have to speak if we do not want to. We don't even have to tell people our names. We can simply say something like, "I pass. I'm just here to listen and learn." It's that easy.

It's a safe environment because when we tell our story, no one will interrupt us with advice on what we should do. We can simply say what we need to say, as long as it is brief and takes a short amount of time so others may speak as well. Another value of the meeting is to linger after it is over and get phone numbers from people who work the program. Then, when we run into a difficult situation, we have someone to call who can walk us through it using the principles of the program.

People from all walks of life attend Twelve-Step meetings, all genders, all professions and occupations. What we have in common is our desire to find serenity whether or not the addict is in recovery. In meetings, we learn useful tools and slogans that make life easier.

Each meeting has a different "feel" and people are encouraged to attend meetings in different locations to find the ones that feel right for them. In many communities, it's possible to attend several meetings in one day, and many people do that in the beginning of their recovery. To find meeting locations, go to www.al-anon.org. For cocaine addiction, check out www.co-anon.org. Many people find Codependents Anonymous of great help as well, at www.coda.org. Free publications can also be downloaded from these sites.

There are many other Twelve-Step programs, in addition to these. If you search, you will find the one that is right for you.

## What is a sponsor?

In his book *Broken*, William Cope Moyers writes, "Every newcomer in AA is told to get a sponsor, somebody who has been sober and in the program for an extended period of time. A sponsor is really a teacher who has 'been there and done that' and who is willing to share his or her experience with others" (p. 212).

In finding a sponsor, people are encouraged to find a person who "says what you like and seems to have found the solutions you seek." Sponsors have different ways of working with their *sponsees* (the person being sponsored), but in general, they make themselves available to take phone calls or have lunch/coffee for the purpose of finding out how things are going and making recommendations for working a healthy program of recovery, which includes working the Twelve Steps.

The sponsor/sponsee relationship is confidential.

## Should I tell the addict to call a sponsor or call the sponsor myself when I see something going on?

Calling the sponsor is often the first response we want to make because we have a tendency to watch the addict's every move and make judgments. Remember that the addict needs time to integrate the information and tools learned at the treatment center. Addicts may not respond or behave the way you think they should, but that does not mean they aren't doing anything.

Our loved one's recovery program was extensive and our loved one was given the tools to continue recovery. It is his or her choice how to work the program. Remember, it's not our responsibility. We cannot control our loved one's recovery. The best way to respond is to share our feelings by saying something like:

* I am concerned that....
* I feel...when you....
* It seems to me that....

## Why does the Twelve-Step program promote rigorous honesty?

Don't I have to lie sometimes to protect my children/spouse/parent from the truth? Since the goal of Twelve-Step programs is for people to be "happy, joyous, and free," rigorous honesty is non-negotiable. A frequently heard slogan in recovery programs is, "Our secrets make us sick."

We can test this by telling someone we trust the whole truth about something we have been trying to hide or disguise. How do we feel after having revealed the secret? *Relieved.*

Anyone who believes he or she has to lie to protect someone else may be practicing self-centeredness (we're in the center, trying to direct other people's behavior and outcomes). Our responsibility to ourselves and to other people is to tell the truth. That's how we build trust with each other.

To lie in order to protect someone is saying we do not believe he or she is worthy to hear the truth. It's an act of disrespect and negation.

## What does Higher Power mean? There's only <u>one</u> God, right?

When we set an alarm clock, we are giving permission for that alarm to be our higher power. Without it, we might oversleep, miss important appointments, and create unnecessary chaos in our lives. So the alarm clock is a higher power than we are. This is our choice.

The Internal Revenue Service is a higher power. There are tax deadlines and money that must be paid. It's the law. Most of us recognize that we are not greater than the IRS, and we meet our responsibilities. If we don't, we are inviting unnecessary conflict and chaos into our lives. Still, it is a choice.

So a Higher Power is what we submit to. We choose to obey it because it makes our lives better than they would be if we defied it.

The word "God" has such different definitions for different people. Some people think of God and a "Higher Power" as one and the same. It works for them. For other people, God has been represented to be angry and vengeful, two emotions that are not helpful in recovery, so it may be better to think of a Higher Power that is apart from the God they learned about in a religious context. This will help them to establish a loving relationship with a power greater than themselves: a power that wants the best for them. This Higher Power might even be the Twelve Steps.

> Once I heard a man in an Al-Anon meeting—a college professor—struggle with the concept of a Higher Power. He finally came to the conclusion that, at least for the time being, the Al-Anon group would be his Higher Power. That is, he would follow the group guidelines instead of trying to figure everything out on his own, using mental processes. This approach worked for him until, through the spiritual processes of the program, he could establish a loving relationship with his own Higher Power.

Most of us believe there is some power in the universe that is greater than we are. We might refer to it as "The Universe" or "Great Spirit," or simply "Love." *In the treatment program I was in, we were asked to define "Higher Power." There were thirty-two of us in the session and there were thirty-two different answers. Our Higher Power is what we are* willing to turn our will and our life over to, if only for a moment. It is a matter of *faith*, not belief.

Once we turn our lives over to a Higher Power (Steps 1-3 of the Twelve-Step program), then we are ready to work the steps. In this process, it's helpful to follow a discipline each day. *The Big Book of Alcoholics Anonymous* has a process that's useful for anyone:

> "As we go through the day, we pause, when agitated or doubtful, and ask for the right thought or action. We constantly remind ourselves that we are no longer running the show, humbly saying to ourselves many times each day 'Thy will be done.' We are then in much less danger of excitement, fear, anger, worry, self-pity, or foolish decisions. We become much more efficient. We do not tire so easily, for we are not burning up energy foolishly as we did when we were trying to arrange life to suit ourselves. It works—it really does." (p. 87-88)

Here's a story of a woman's struggle to identify and accept her Higher Power

> Near the end of our twenty-eight-day treatment, my roommate stormed into the room. I was sitting on the deck, overlooking a beautiful stream and enjoying the cool spring day. She had just come from a session with her counselors, and she was agitated: "They say I can't leave until I find my Higher Power." Since I didn't know how to respond, I said nothing. I just continued to sit there and enjoy the day. She came out onto the deck and sat beside me. For many minutes, we simply sat in silence.
>
> Then she straightened as if with a sudden realization, and said, "That's it."
> "That's what?" I asked.
> There was a long pause.
> "Isn't there a scripture that talks about being still?" she asked.
> "Be still, and know that I am God," I remembered.
> "Yes. That's it."
> In that moment of quiet, my roommate had found her Higher Power.

## What if you don't believe in God? Can you still work a Twelve-Step program?

Yes. The most important thing about a Twelve-Step program is willingness. By the time we get to a Twelve-Step program, we have probably become aware that some things in life are beyond our ability to understand or fix, and we are willing to try something else.

Certain disciplines must be followed in order to be good at life. Just as athletes submit themselves to the discipline of training programs and practice in order to achieve their goals, so those of us in Twelve-Step programs submit ourselves to the discipline of those steps. For an athlete, this discipline means saying "no" to certain foods and "yes" to daily exercise and conditioning. It means doing what the coaches say without resisting. For a Twelve-Stepper, this discipline means saying "no" to emotional outbursts when anxiety strikes and learning to stay in serenity through saying the Serenity Prayer, reading helpful literature, or calling a sponsor for advice. It means following the program without question.

The only requirement for working a Twelve-Step program is willingness. And no one does it perfectly. The mantra is *"progress, not perfection."*

"Each of us is born with the potential for the unfolding of our true self. When you deviate from the truth, you are interfering with the intention of something greater than you are—call it nature or a higher power. As a result, you develop discomfort."

~ Author Unknown

| **7** | **Accessing the Authentic Self—<br>Relationship with God Inventory** |

Being authentic is a journey of acknowledging that we are powerful spiritual beings and co-creators with God. When we remember this truth, we move away from endless negative mind chatter and move directly into our hearts. This space is where our true essence, our knowing, resides. When we align our hearts with God, we ask God to help us see ourselves as God sees us, without any judgment or expectations.

When we live authentically, we act on the guidance we receive, even if our egos or personalities begin to question that guidance. Trusting our guidance is essential. Always remember: what we need to know and do will be revealed to us with perfect timing.

Here is an exercise to help you access the authentic self.

---

1. What is your understanding of God/Higher Power now?




---

2. Do you experience God's/Higher Power's presence in your life?

**3. Describe your relationship with God/Higher Power**

...Growing up

...Today

**4. When have you felt the presence of God/Higher Power manifesting in your life?**

**5. What would it take for you to experience that presence now?**

**6. Do you trust God/Higher Power? Describe.**

**7. What is your understanding of God's will for you? Describe.**

**8. If you do believe in God/Higher Power, what do you believe in and what do you trust?**

## Trust

Often, we feel afraid or overwhelmed with what is going on in our lives. We respond with fear, panic, helplessness, and distrust. We may not trust ourselves or our Higher Power/God, resorting to old controlling behaviors. We can deal with the need to control by approaching our fear. We deal with fear by being honest with ourselves about our fear, by trusting ourselves, trusting our Higher Power, and trusting the process we call recovery.

We trust that when things don't seem to work out the way we want, God has a better plan for us. We can trust ourselves to know where we need to go, what to say, what to do, what to know, what to be. We trust in God's guidance, and we respond to that guidance through listening and responding.

Webster's Dictionary defines trust as:

- Reliance on Integrity
- Strength and ability of a person
- Confidence / Confident expectation
- Hope

Trust is a mixture of:

- Faith
- Willingness
- Humility / Vulnerability
- Courage to take risks

Trust is the beginning of letting go of the unrealistic notion of control.
Trust is a paradigm: The glass is half-full vs. the glass is half-empty.
Trust is the vision beyond appearances.

Here is an exercise for dealing with your own trust issues:

1.  **Write all your Trust issues:**


2.  **Who and what do you mistrust and why?**

3.  Who and what do you truly trust?

4.  Do you trust yourself? (Describe how and why.)

5.  What would you need to be and do in order to feel trustworthy?

6.    **What would others need to be and do in order for you to trust them?**

## Boundaries

We are often told we need to create boundaries, but the concept can be difficult, especially since families marked by addiction and codependence have an absence of them.

What Is A Boundary?

- It is a line that marks a limit not to be crossed.

- It is a border, not to be entered or used without permission.

- It is a safety guideline.

- It is what defines us as unique and individual.

What Is The Role Of Boundaries?

- Boundaries help us to take care of ourselves by setting limits.

- Boundaries allow us to get close to others when it is appropriate.

- Boundaries help us to maintain our distance when we might be harmed or taken advantage of by getting too close.

- Boundaries help us protect ourselves from abuse while we pave the way to achieving true intimacy.

- Boundaries determine where we start and end—and where the other person starts.

- Boundaries are limits we need to set in relationships.

- Boundaries allow us to separate our own thoughts and feelings from those of others.

- Boundaries help us develop a strong sense of responsibility for what we think, feel, and do.

- Boundaries help us develop a strong and healthy sense of self.

## Types of Boundaries and Guidelines

Boundaries define our uniqueness and need for respect and safety:

- **Physical boundaries:** your space, privacy, possessions, need for hygiene and order
- **Emotional boundaries:** your feelings, emotions, perceptions, intuitions, love, trust, secrets, promises, commitments, needs, friendships, relationships
- **Intellectual Boundaries:** your ideas, thoughts, perceptions, opinions, priorities and preferences
- **Sexual Boundaries:** your body, sexual organs, sensuality, sexual expression, fidelity, sexual safety
- **Financial Boundaries:** financial integrity and trustworthiness, financial responsibility and accountability, financial promises, commitments and promises honored
- **Spiritual Boundaries:** Respect for your spiritual beliefs and practices, freedom of spiritual beliefs, your values and morals
- **Social Boundaries:** Choice of friends, common friends, belonging to a recovering community (AA or Al-Anon), respect for your friends
- **Cultural Boundaries:** Respect and courtesy for your origins, traditions, and values; respect for family traditions without ridicule
- **Political Boundaries:** Respect and understanding of your political beliefs, choices, and affiliations

## Boundaries Can Be Spoken or Unspoken, Overt Or Covert!

The addict and his/her family in their co-dependent dysfunction have a hard time setting healthy boundaries.

In some families, the boundaries are rigid, unbending, and loudly stated with severe consequences if crossed.

In other families, the boundaries are walls behind which members hide to avoid intimacy. Enmeshment is the order of the day, and no one knows where the boundaries begin or end.

Families where the boundaries are unspoken play the Assuming/Interpreting game. You are supposed to know what others expect from you. You are not allowed to voice your needs and opinions but expected to follow an invisible pattern of conduct.

There is also the family that hides the boundaries under the disguise of "don't want to hurt your feelings"...followed by a guilt trip!

And then there are families with nonexistent boundaries… a free-for-all with a sense of being out of control. No guidelines, no rules, no expectations—just confusion, creating people who will look in life for structure, but will not be able to fit into it.

In an addict's family, the emotional boundaries are the hardest to set and respect, as the emotional charge with which they are approached usually contains all the unspoken frustrations, anger, violations, broken promises, etc. Thus, the past gets constantly projected into the future.

## Emotional Boundaries Define the Self

We are unique beings composed of individual ideas, feelings, values, expressions, and perspectives. We are truly unique. Emotional boundaries allow us to protect our uniqueness.

## What Strengthens Our Emotional Boundaries?

- The freedom to say "no"
- Understanding and respect for our feelings
- Being heard and accepted in our differences
- Being supported in our personal process and development
- Being allowed freedom of expression
- Being empowered in our uniqueness
- Being in a mature environment that is not threatened by our uniqueness

## What Harms Emotional Boundaries?

- Being ridiculed, humiliated, and put down
- Being treated with sarcasm, mockery, and belittling comments
- Name calling and/or any kind of abuse
- Stifling and dishonest communication
- Smothering in the name of love
- Insistence on conformity
- Broken promises and lies
- Unfairness and arbitrariness
- Judgments, criticism, and blame
- The need to overpower and dominate

## Why Do I Need Healthy Boundaries?

- Unhealthy and dysfunctional boundaries are rigid, demanding, disrespectful, confusing, unfair, or non-existent.

- *Healthy boundaries* are flexible, inclusive, clear, and safe. They promote a healthy sense of self and one's uniqueness and are respectful of others.

- Boundaries are for us, and not for the addict/alcoholic or any other person. They define what we are willing to accept. We do not have to accept unacceptable behavior, so it's good to get clear on what acceptable behavior looks like.

## Setting an Effective Boundary

The following story portrays one wife's success with boundary setting:

> My husband was sober off-and-on for about five years. He would be fine for a while, and then he would start drinking again, not coming home until 2 a.m. or even later. I had a full-time job and small children. I needed my sleep, which was being disturbed by his behavior.
>
> With the help of Al-Anon, I set a boundary. I told him not to come home drunk in the middle of the night because I needed my sleep. After I told him this, he did it again. I realized I had to take action. At the time, I couldn't afford to change the lock, and the best solution I could think of was to put Scotch tape over the keyhole. It worked. When he came home in the wee hours of the morning, he was so drunk that he couldn't figure out how to open the door.
>
> The next morning, as I pulled out of the garage with the children, there he was, asleep in his car in the driveway. My son asked what was wrong with Dad. "He isn't feeling well" was my reply. That was almost twenty years ago, and he has been sober ever since. In fact, we just celebrated our thirty-fifth wedding anniversary. I am so grateful for the wonderful Al-Anon members who loved and encouraged me in those early days until I learned enough to take action that was right for me.

## The Difference between a Boundary and a Wall

Boundaries are healthy, but walls aren't. Here's a story from one mother about when she discovered how to scale back from a wall to more healthy boundaries:

> When my son came home from treatment, my husband and I got help for ourselves. The most important thing I learned was the difference between setting a boundary and building a wall. I learned to tell my son, without anger or forcefulness, what I needed in order for us to successfully live together. I didn't raise my voice.
>
> A boundary isn't very tall; it's just a line. What I used to do was put up a thick, impenetrable wall. I didn't tell him what I needed; instead, I "laid down the law," with an attitude of "You do this because I say so. You have to do it because I'm your mother." Well, that didn't get the results I wanted. Instead, it threw my son and me into this sick game where each of us was trying to make the other do what we wanted.
>
> I've learned that when I'm unsure, worried, scared, and upset, my ego is in charge. I've learned to get calm so that the true, authentic self within me can speak.
>
> My son recently said, "You're no fun anymore." What he means was that he can't manipulate me anymore. And I don't try to manipulate him, either.
>
> Recently, after not quite a year of sobriety, he started drinking again. When he called to tell me, I was calm. My husband and I paid for his treatment; he knows what to do, and he has some tools when he decides to get sober. I've done my part; now it's up to him. I'm very grateful that he told me the truth, and I'm respecting him to figure out what is best for him. This is my boundary.

## What to Do With Unacceptable Behavior

If we think our alcoholic/addicted loved one is being returned to us as perfect, we need to think again. Who among us is perfect? Addictions are accompanied by behaviors like lying, being self-centered, not considering other people, and being egotistical.

Our loved one is learning a new way to live, and as he or she is learning, those old behaviors resurface from time to time. When we see one of these behaviors, we need to turn our eyes inward. *If you spot it, you've got it.* We ask ourselves, "How am I being inconsiderate?" The part of the process is to ask God to remove that character defect from within us. Call someone in the Al-Anon program and work a Fourth Step, which requires a searching and fearless moral inventory, as soon as you can.

This is a proven way to keep your love for the addict healthy. We cannot and do not help by pointing out the addict's flaws. We must keep the focus on ourselves. We must draw the boundary between what is and what is not our personal responsibility.

## What Is My Circle Of Influence And Personal Responsibility?

- My INNER and OUTER awareness
- My INNER awareness includes: my beliefs, thoughts, feelings, decisions, choices, experiences, needs, wants, and unconscious material
- My OUTER awareness includes: my perceptions, behaviors, actions, and reactions

*IT IS MY RESPONSIBILITY TO MAKE MY LIFE*
*SUCCESSFUL AND JOYFUL.*

## What is *Not* In My Circle of Influence and is Not My Responsibility?

- Other people's INNER awareness: their beliefs, thoughts, feelings, decisions, choices, experiences, needs and wants, and unconscious material.
- Other people's OUTER awareness: their perceptions, behaviors, actions, and reactions

*IT IS THEIR RESPONSIBILITY TO MAKE THEIR LIVES*
*SUCCESSFUL AND JOYFUL.*

| 8 | # Questions About Your Relationship with the Addict |
|---|---|

## What's the difference between *good* enabling and *bad* enabling?

One of the definitions of *enable* is "to strengthen." So in issues of enabling, it's good to ask, "What behavior am I strengthening?" Needless to say, as loved ones of alcoholics and addicts, we want to strengthen behaviors that are life-giving and not those that feed the addiction.

In his book *Broken*, William Cope Moyers, son of noted journalist Bill Moyers, tells the story of getting out of treatment for his cocaine addiction and going home to a stack of unpaid bills and a wife who was about to divorce him. To help him out with his bills, his parents gave him $5,000, which he promptly took to his drug dealer and continued to spend on cocaine until the money was all gone. Unwittingly, his parents *strengthened* his ability to buy drugs, while his debts went unpaid. Even the intelligent and revered Bill Moyers did not realize he was *enabling* his son's addiction.

Addiction, according to *The Big Book of Alcoholics Anonymous*, is "cunning, baffling, and powerful." As loved ones, we sometimes confuse our desire for the addict's behavior with the actual behavior. We may see what we want to believe rather than what is. Loved ones do not want to believe this disease is so powerful that it can cause a child to betray his parents or a husband to betray his wife or a mother to betray her child. We don't understand that the addiction is so powerful that the addict will do anything to get the drug the addiction craves. And we desperately want to believe that twenty-eight to ninety or more days in treatment will actually *cure* our loved one, just as if the addict had a curable disease and had paid for the medical treatment that will end the problem. We want to be rid of the problem.

Addiction is not curable. But it responds well to treatment. Sobriety—even happiness— can be maintained for a lifetime if the addict continues to apply the principles of the program and grow, as *The Big Book* says, "along spiritual lines."

If we want to *enable* healthy, independent living, we will say something like, "I'm not giving you any money. In the past, you haven't used what I've given you to serve your best interests, and I see no evidence now that you can spend money well. I have faith that you will figure out what you need to do. I love you." And leave it at that. These words will be spoken from a loving, kind state of mind. Here's how one person came to understand the true dangers of enabling:

> During family week at a treatment center, I listened to the heart-wrenching voice of a father who had bailed his son out of jail time-after-time. As he told the story, the father said, "I love him to death."
>
> The wise facilitator interrupted. "Precisely. Your so-called love will send him to his death if you don't stop."

The father's actions, in the name of love, *enabled* the son to keep on doing what he was doing, knowing his father would always come to bail him out—a very misguided sense of what love is. What is the alternative? Leave the addict alone to accept the consequences of his actions. This choice *enables* responsibility and maturity on our part.

Here's a metaphor that helps to understand this concept:

> Once an observer watched a butterfly trying to emerge from a cocoon. Touched by the mighty struggle, he decided to help the butterfly by tearing the cocoon, setting it free to fly. But the butterfly didn't fly. Instead, it lay limply in the torn cocoon, fluttered a bit, and eventually died on the branch. Its wings needed the struggle of emerging from the cocoon to gain the strength needed for flight.

The observer's desire to help got the best of him, and he freed the butterfly without realizing his actions would ultimately bring harm. If we feel we "love someone to death," we have to consider what we're really saying. *Do I love that person so much I'm going to keep on doing what I'm doing, regardless of the outcome?* If so, is that really love? Or is it a selfish desire on our part not to change? Or a stubborn refusal to accept the truth? One wife whose husband finally got sober tells this story from her early experience with him in recovery:

> My mother-in-law was my husband's enabler. When I threw him out of the house, she let him stay with her. When he was on the streets, she gave him money. She paid his debts. She believed everything he told her. For instance, he told her he needed $100 to go to the doctor. She gave it to him. Of course, he used it to buy drugs.

> Addiction loves its drugs of choice above all else. More than wives. More than husbands. More than children. More than parents or friends. It will do anything, including lying and stealing from people who love the addict, to keep using the drugs. And it lies to the addict about what it is really doing. What starts the process of setting people free from addiction is telling them the truth with love and leaving them alone to deal with the consequences.

## Should I get rid of the alcohol in the house?

The best answer is to ask how the addict feels about it. In some cases, the addict may feel it would be best not to have access to the alcohol. However, it's important to know that if the addict is going to drink, he or she will, regardless of whether you keep alcohol in the house.

## Why is it important to give up control?

Here are two stories that will help illustrate the answer to this question.

### First Story

When my brother came out of recovery, my sister was eager for him to have a "normal" life. He had nothing; he was bankrupt and going to school to learn a new career. My sister decided to buy him a cell phone. When he heard her plans, he said, "No. Don't do that. I can use a pay phone."

His new job was driving a truck, and my sister's notion was that she needed to know where he was. She would be frightened if he were out of reach by phone. So, over his objections, she bought him a cell phone and was then furious with him when he went way over on his allotted minutes, and she had to pay his big telephone bill.

But whose fault was it, really? All along, he told her he did not want a cell phone, and she did not respect his request. She was trying to control this part of his life in order to soothe herself, and it ended badly for both of them.

### Second Story

My business partner and best friend for twenty years was an alcoholic. She was a functioning alcoholic, and she was a lot of fun when she was drinking. In fact, I drank with her.

But over time, that changed. She started coming to work drunk, and she was unmanageable. I turned into a controlling bitch. The more she drank, the more I tried to control. I've been told my whole life that I'm a control freak; I'm just now getting to understand why it's not good. It's not good because it turns me into an uptight, clenched, unpleasant, unhappy person. When I try to make things perfect, I can't be happy because that's impossible.

Eventually my friend tried to commit suicide and was given mandatory rehab (which I think is an oxymoron). She hated AA and refused to go. When she got out of treatment, she started drinking again immediately. She walked away from our business, abandoned everything, and moved back home with her mother.

Because of my experience with my friend, I've come to realize that all of my aunts and uncles are alcoholics, as well as my ex-husband and every other man with whom I've ever had a serious relationship. Also, my son, who lives with me, has addiction problems.

In Al-Anon, I'm learning to keep the focus on myself. I'm reading the daily meditations, and I'm concentrating on my own healing. I've also started going back to church.

All this time, I didn't even know I had a problem. I thought I knew what was right, and I was very frustrated that other people couldn't understand it. Now I understand that I'm not God. The disease of alcoholism/addiction is cunning, baffling, powerful, and beyond my ability to control. So I'm letting go.

> When you try to control things that are beyond your control—like the behavior of another person—you are putting yourself in the place of God. You are not God. When you try to control, you are taking up the space that belongs to God. That's why we say "Let go and let God."

## What is denial (minimizing/discounting/rationalizing)?

Simply stated, denial is refusing to acknowledge the truth. It can take the form of making excuses for one's own or someone else's behavior. It's pretending that all is well when, in reality, life is chaotic. Here's a real-life example:

> When I arrived for Thanksgiving dinner, the first thing my mother said to me was, "Please go pick up your brother." Well, I knew he had been drinking and drugging for days, hadn't slept, and would probably throw up in my car. So I refused, and someone else went to get him.
>
> No sooner had we sat down to dinner than my brother fell face-forward into his plate. I got up and left.

In this story, the mother was determined to have a "normal" Thanksgiving dinner. Not acknowledging the seriousness of her son's condition, she was not able to have respect for the impact his drunken presence would have on other members of the family. This mother's behavior is a classic example of denial.

Denial is rooted in a strong desire to avoid confrontation. It's living a lie. The longer denial exists in a family, the longer the addict's behavior will continue to sabotage the family dynamics and wreak havoc in family members' lives.

### What should I look for if I think my loved one is using?

Looking for ways to have peace within ourselves is essential. We need to work our own Twelve-Step program. This question reveals an *other-focused* perspective. We need to keep the focus on ourselves, and let our loved one take care of his or her own business.

### How do I support loved ones when they continue to relapse?

Here's story of a relapse from the wife's perspective:

My husband has used cocaine for as long as I've known him—twenty years. When we married, we both used. I thought he would outgrow it. Instead, I was the one who outgrew it. He didn't. It was easy for me to ignore his addiction because he wasn't mean to me. In fact, I was the one who went ballistic. Once I beat a hole in the wall with a hammer, trying to get to him in a locked bedroom and stop him from using. I even hit him. So I was the crazy one!

Eventually, he was arrested for using illegal drugs. He underwent various kinds of treatment through the years. His last treatment was a twenty-eight day program, and I really hoped it would be the end of his using. But within just a few weeks out of treatment, he used again. This time, I asked him to move out—for the first time. Subsequently, he got arrested and is in jail right now, awaiting trial.

The last time I spoke with him, he asked me whether I was going to divorce him. I said, "I don't know, and I'm not ready to make that decision right now. There's way too much else for me to think about."

In Al-Anon and Co-Anon, I've learned to keep the focus on myself and do what is right for me, regardless of what he says or does. My fear of not being able to make it financially without him is fading, and I feel emotionally stable. I also know that I don't have to tackle all my problems at once; I just have to do the next right thing.

## How can I learn to communicate with my child/spouse/parent better?

The most important thing about communication is our own emotional state during the conversation. Those of us who have lived with addiction have turned our emotions off. We're almost like zombies, "zoned out" so we cannot be hurt again. Occasionally, we explode with anger, throw a fit, and then feel better for a while until our unacknowledged emotions build to the breaking point again.

We need to start paying attention to the emotion that lies underneath our communication with our child/spouse/parent. *Am I angry? Sad? Worried? Or am I Kind? Considerate? Forgiving?*

It's the *emotion* that people hear, the tone in our voice, not the words. The best advice is not to speak to a loved one when we are angry. We must process the anger, make a searching and fearless moral inventory (i.e., the Fourth Step) with a sponsor, and get to the willingness to forgive before we broach a sensitive topic with a loved one.

In particular, you must not nag. Nagging is defined as making the same request more than once. People, not only addicts, dislike this; nagging makes them tune us out, which makes our chance of communicating even less.

Author Greg Baer says that when we speak in anger, the message the other person receives is that we do not love him or her. To build a loving relationship, we must put more love into it. So a guiding question for conversations with loved ones is, "What would love do?" or "How may I be most loving and respectful, and at the same time, say what is right for me?"

What finally brings many addicts into recovery is a nonjudgmental, loving confrontation from someone they love. Something as simple as, "No, son. It's not okay. Not this time."

In communicating with people we love, we must search for our own intent. Are we trying to manipulate? If so, then we must not say it. Are we bribing? If so, then we must keep our mouths shut. Are we pointing out their faults? Forget it; we all have them, and we won't help by pointing theirs out. We have to be honest with ourselves about our true motives.

> "They may forget what you said, but they will never forget how you made them feel."
>
> — Carl W. Buechner

<table>
<tr><td>**9**</td><td></td></tr>
</table>

# Success Stories

Stories of people who have overcome addiction are inspiring and help remind both the addict and the co-addict family members that a better day is possible. Offered here are several success stories to remind people that change is possible and recovery can lead to a bright new tomorrow.

## Success Story #1

The first success story is told from both the addicted mother's point of view, and then her daughter's point of view.

### A Mother's Story

From eighth grade to age thirty, I was a binge drinker. That means I did not drink every day; I only drank to party, and when I drank, I blacked out. Although I never remembered a thing, I was the life of the party. I never got arrested for drunk driving, but I did lose several bartending jobs because I was drinking on the job.

Growing up, I never felt like I fit in. Although I had five brothers and two sisters, I felt like an only child because I had a different mother from my siblings. I did not look like anyone else in my family. In my teenage years, I ran away from home a lot. When I made a mistake, my parents would ground me, so I just ran away.

Dad, who was a practicing alcoholic, was determined to tame me. Once he took me to the police and said, "She's incorrigible. Do something with her." Well, they put me in a home for runaways, and I just ran away again. Eventually, I met a boy two years older than me—I was sixteen at the time—who was a violent alcoholic. With him, I experienced physical and sexual abuse.

My parents, especially my stepmother, did everything they could think of to help me. My stepmom is a loving, nurturing person. She started going to Al-Anon when I was sixteen, and our family—because of my behavior—went through a lot of counseling. Once in a visit with her counselor, my stepmom said, "Why am I doing this? No one is getting sober." The counselor wisely responded, "Because someday somebody will get sober, and you want to be ready for them." This bit of hope kept her going.

At the age of thirty, I stopped drinking. That was October of 1988. But it wasn't until the following March that I gave up pot and speed. I thought giving up alcohol was enough; I was going to AA. But I was having recurring dreams of black spirits chasing me, and I prayed to God to tell me what to do.

At about the same time, a counselor asked me to participate in an intervention on my husband's cousin. That experience led me to the employee assistance program through my husband's employer, and then to treatment.

At that time, my family was my Higher Power. I went to treatment to save my family. I stayed in treatment for ninety days. I was a tough case because I simply would not do what they told me to do. I resisted opening up. But finally, I did it, and I went back home to the life of my dreams.

I had told my husband I would be happy if I had a nice home with a swimming pool in the backyard and a Jeep. He gave me everything I asked for. At age thirty-nine, I was excited to turn forty. My life was awesome, and I still loved my husband. I was active in my daughter's school—PTA officer, talent shows, booster clubs.

But then, after twelve years of sobriety, I started drinking again. I was on vacation with my family in Canada. We were out on a boat, and I reached into the cooler for a bottle of water. Instead, I grasped a can of beer and simply opened it and started drinking. This happened the summer after my daughter left home.

Then I realized I didn't want to go home. I wasn't happy in my marriage. At forty-two, I divorced, and for two years I drank.

My first sobriety was for my family; my second sobriety was for me. Two things made me go back into AA and recovery. First was the shame of waking up from a blackout in an alley with a man I didn't know. The second was that someone I was dating was court-ordered to go to AA. From him, I started hearing the promises of AA (*The Big Book of Alcoholics Anonymous* p. 83-84). I wanted what the promises offered and the blessing of the program. I knew my life could be better.

While she was growing up, my daughter got exposed to things that weren't good for her. She even got her own alarm clock because she couldn't rely on me to wake her up for school in the morning. She didn't bring friends home. She couldn't count on me.

For families of alcoholics, I have two bits of advice:

Lock the door and keep it locked. Don't let us back in. We'll taunt you with words like, "Oh, you like me when I'm sober and not when I'm drunk." We'll do anything to try to keep you and keep on drinking. Force us to make a choice.

Get a support group. I'll always be grateful that my stepmom went to Al-Anon. I think it helped. The counselor was right. One of us DID get sober. That was me. And she was ready for me.

## Her Daughter's Story

I don't remember much until around age five or six. We were living in a house full of construction workers, and from Friday through Sunday it was party time. I poured the beer. I was the bartender, and I got tips.

Mom calls me "Babydoll." That's what I was—her baby doll. She took me everywhere, like little girls do with their baby dolls. I knew it was wrong, but I also knew I would get tips.

Mom was a happy drunk, not abusive at all. I was never left uncared for. I remember on my seventh birthday she stayed up on speed for two days, getting ready for my party. Then she crashed and slept for two days. Dad was there, but I learned to make it without Mom. I became very self-sufficient and independent. I made my own breakfast. I got myself to school.

Only once do I remember her getting physical with me. When I was five or six, we spent the night at her dealer's house. The next morning, I couldn't find my shoe. She became so angry with me that she picked me up by my ear. It hurt so bad. I saw the horrified look in her eyes when she realized what she was doing. She put me down and walked away.

Throughout these years, I knew something was wrong. I'd hear her crying on the phone, but I was too young to understand about addiction.

When I was six years old, Mom went into treatment. It was traumatic for me. She told me she was sick and could not get well by herself. She had to go away so that she could be a better mom. I wasn't happy to hear this. I asked, "But who will take care of me?!" I told her not to go. No. It was not all right with me.

Then one day when I came home from school, my stepdad—whom I had never been close to—was there, sitting on the couch. I said, "Where's Mom?" He said, "She's gone away to get well." And he was crying. I dropped my backpack and flung myself on the couch beside him. For about half an hour, we cried in each other's arms. This was bonding time for us. From that time on, he was my dad.

I was so excited when she came home. With some of my friends and the help of my grandma, I put on a puppet show to welcome her home. I remember her saying to me, "You need to be a little girl. Stop trying to take care of Mom."

She was a different mom. All of a sudden, now out of treatment, she became involved in my life. She joined PTA—not just as a parent, but she was an officer, and involved full force. It felt almost like she traded one addiction for another. At school, she was almost more popular than me.

Then she fell off the wagon. On a trip to Canada, she got out of hand, and it was apparent that there was still a problem. You wouldn't have known she had experienced one minute of sobriety from the way she acted. This event let me realize that addiction is not curable; you have to keep working at it. It's a progressive disease.

Then came the Fourth of July. We were together at a joint on the lake, watching the fireworks. Mom got into a fight with some guy, and I walked her home to the boat where she was living. I put her to bed and went back to be with my friends.

After the fireworks, my friends and I decided to go swimming. I figured Mom was asleep, so we could swim off the boat, and we started walking to the boat. As we got close, I saw Mom, naked. She had been skinny dipping with some guy. I was so ashamed. I pleaded with my friends not to look, and we got out of there.

Later, when she said, "I'm so sorry, Babydoll," I replied, "I know, but it's not enough. It's embarrassing." This was the first time I told her how her drinking affected me. I was about twenty-two years old.

About six weeks later, she got sober again. She's been sober ever since.

I feel blessed. God had to be carrying Mom through all these ordeals. And I always felt safe. I never felt abandoned or that my mom did a bad job.

The most traumatic time for me was when Mom and Dad split up, when I was nineteen. In my family, I was always the common denominator. When my family fell apart, I fell apart. I was so angry at Mom. I resented her for breaking up my foundation. I started having panic attacks. Mom and Dad got counseling for me, and now when I get anxious, I know how to calm down.

My greatest fear these days is that I am like my mom. Every time I order a second glass of wine, I wonder whether I'm overdoing it. And my upbringing has affected my relationship with men. I don't want to leave my man after nineteen years. It's still hard for me to understand why Mom did that. I want to find someone I can stay with forever. I did find someone like that once, and I ran away.

But God is doing for me what I cannot do for myself. My aunt tells me I'm nothing like my mom. When my mom was my age (twenty-eight), she had spent years drinking and drugging, was divorced, and had a child. I've done none of those things, so I hope I can love someone the way she couldn't.

## Success Story #2

What do you do when you don't know what to do? I was from a fundamentalist religious family. I didn't believe I was an alcoholic because I had money, a car, a house, a family. I wasn't a lowlife scumbag. I was from a good family. That's how little I knew about alcoholism.

After our baby was born, I nursed for six weeks. When that was over, I turned to pills and alcohol to ease my anxiety. I would get up at midnight with the baby, and while I changed and fed him, I'd have a glass of wine, or two.

Our marriage was a disaster; my husband kept trying to control what I did. He took my keys away; he took the money away. He would do anything to make me stop drinking. In the process, he was mentally, physically, and emotionally abusive to me. Because of my religion, I thought I had to stay with him.

Finally, I ended up in treatment. At the end of the month, my husband picked me up, and on the way home, told me he was divorcing me and taking the baby. This was more than I could handle, so I started drinking again.

I got an apartment, and for the first time in my life, I was alone. There was no one to monitor my activities or tell me what to do.

What led to my sobriety was an automobile accident. I wrecked a brand new Land Rover and ended up in the hospital. Since there was no one else, a social worker came to take me home. She talked to me about alcoholism in a nonjudgmental, kind way. She gave me some pamphlets with telephone numbers. I started going to AA, and I haven't had a drink since. That was two years ago.

My message to families is this: Educate yourselves and understand that this disease is an allergy of the body and an obsession of the mind. It is real. Once you understand it, you know someone cannot "just stop drinking." Alcoholism is not a dirty word, but it is deadly.

Because of alcoholism, all I had left was God. And God is all I need. Sometimes in treatment, people try to cram so much information into their heads. They try so hard to figure it out and get it right—fix themselves. Really, all it takes is God—to acknowledge that I am powerless over alcohol, to believe that a power greater than me can restore me to sanity, and to make a decision to turn my will and my life over to the care of God, as I understand Him.

I've heard people say, "Don't stop drinking for other people. Do it for yourself." Honestly, some days I decide not to drink because of my son. Those days, I stay sober for him. I want to be a good mom. That's okay. It takes whatever it takes—one day at a time.

My mother thinks I'm cured. She tries to put me on a pedestal. That's naïve on her part and not helpful to me. I know my sobriety is just one day at a time, and the only thing that keeps me sober is staying spiritually fit and attending AA meetings *that are focused on solutions, where I learn from other alcoholics what works.*

# Part II:
# Changing Yourself

Recovery is not for the people who need it.
It's not even for the people who want it.
It's for the people who DO it.
Trace it.
Face it.
Erase it.
Replace it.

Author Unknown

# 10 Making the Changes in Your Life First

One woman's story about the Fourth Step and why it matters:

When I was a teenager, my family had a kitchen stove with one burner that could be lowered so that a deep pot fit into the space. Mother used to make vegetable beef soup in that pot.

I loved Mother's vegetable beef soup, but I hated the cleanup afterward, which was my job. So one evening, I decided I would just put the lid on that pot of leftover soup, clean neatly around it with the dishcloth so it looked clean from the outside, and leave it there.

Weeks went by, and Mother said nothing about the leftover pot of soup. I wondered whether she had cleaned it, and if so, why I hadn't gotten a tongue-lashing for not finishing the job.

Finally, my curiosity got the best of me, and one afternoon, when she was away from home, I lifted the lid. What a mess! She hadn't found it—or, if she had, she had chosen to say nothing. It was still there for me to clean up—only worse now because it had grown green, gray, and orange fuzzy stuff, and it smelled bad. Now I had no choice. It *had* to be cleaned up. So I did it.

My teenage soup pot experience involved the same process as a Fourth Step. Something happens that we choose to "put the lid on"—we don't want to face it at the time, for whatever reason. We hope it will just go away. While we're in this state of denial, things get worse. Since our denial has not succeeded in making the unpleasantness go away, some of us find the courage to "lift the lid." We face the problem. Then we do our part to clean it up. And from that time forward, we do not leave a soup pot unwashed.

In learning to change ourselves, here is the process we follow:

- Remember what you did or left undone. (Trace it.)
- Lift the lid. (Face it.)
- Do all you can to clean it up. (Erase it.)
- From that moment on, clean the soup pot immediately after using it. (Replace it.)

## Taking the Steps to Change

During treatment, the addict may have attended a Twelve-Step program. The Twelve-Step program was first created for overcoming addiction to alcohol, but it has since been used also for other behavioral issues. Basically, its focus is to: "Trust God, clean house [our own life], help others." Before we can help others, in this case the recovering addict who comes home, we need to clean our own house. Trusting God is certainly the first element with which we must come to terms. Whether or not we are religious, Trusting God (Higher Power, or whatever label we wish to put on "it") is fundamental to whether the process will be easy or detrimental.

The American Psychological Association summarizes the process as follows:

- Admitting that one cannot control one's addiction or compulsion;

- Recognizing a greater power that can give strength;

- Examining past errors with the help of a sponsor (experienced member);

- Making amends for these errors;

- Learning to live a new life with a new code of behavior;

- Helping others who suffer from the same addictions or compulsions.

- The Twelve Step Principles: Honesty, Humility, Hope, Purity of Intent, Love

## Honesty is:

- Going into action after having faced the facts about ourselves.

- Facing fear and getting out of it.

- Discernment: we have no right to dump our guilt on others in the name of honesty.

- Knowing our limitations.

- Being in touch with our feelings and needs.

- Respecting our choices and commitments.

- Not imposing our truth on others.

- Evaluating and discerning…not condemning.

- Being objective…not self-righteous.
- Being flexible…not rigid and demanding.
- Being in the now moment—not the past or the future.
- Not having a tendency to be minimized or bragged about.
- Minding our own business.
- Truth, and truth is respect.

**Honesty starts with me being honest with ME.**

**Honesty is Action:**  To admit
          To come to believe

**Dishonesty is Reaction:** To take the stance of spectators who observe, criticize, and condemn others.

## Humility is:

- Listening without the need to top what is said
- Being present and listening without the need to bring the conversation back to self
- Being interested in the other person. Asking questions
- Speaking sentences without *I-Me-Myself*
- Being in a situation where you could say, "See? I told you so!" but not saying it
- The capacity to say "please" and ask for what we need without feeling diminished
- The capacity to be vulnerable…the absence of over-sensitivity
- Having a sense of humor; not taking self so seriously; the capacity to laugh at our own mistakes
- The capacity to learn from children
- The capacity to ask for help and to be a team player
- Teachability and openness of mind and heart
- The capacity to fail, learn from mistakes, and not have all the answers
- The foundation of Step One. Without humility, there is no inner strength to do Step One, which is "Admit we are powerless over alcohol and our lives have become unmanageable. Without humility, there is no progress
- The foundation of Step Two: I can't do it—but God can. I recognize a Higher Power only when I stop *being it*…and that takes humility
- The attitude of Gratitude

## Hope is:

- The opposite of worry—short-term or long-term
- Freedom from fear; it is anticipating with trust, knowing that everybody is okay including me, and knowing that everyone has choices.
- The conviction that everything is changing and evolving; nothing is permanent. Divine Order and Divine Justice prevail.
- Believing that the Divine Plan for my life is now unfolding.
- Having a higher vision.
- Being solution-oriented and miracle-minded.
- Acknowledging circumstances but seeing past them and not buying into them.

Hope that comes from ego is conditional: "I hope, but…" or it is a lot of wishful thinking.

Hope that comes from the identity, our authentic self, is the conviction in our heart that everything is and will be okay regardless of circumstances, in spite of what we might think now, or what our ego would like us to believe.

## Purity of Intent is:

- The pivot of Ego or Identity
- The conscious contact with God
- The basis of Love-Truth—Confidence

We ask, "How *pure* is my *intent*?"—My motives, reasons, purposes, aims, and targets?

If my purpose today is not to be a better human being, chances are my motives will be generated by the *ego* (manipulation, disguised and rationalized selfishness, and the "injustice trap" of self-pity).

But if my purpose today is to be a better human being, regardless of the price to pay, my motives will be generated by the *identity* (honesty, humility, love).

## Love is:

- Not a feeling but a power
- The energy that heals feelings and the power that restores us to sanity
- The substance and essence of you and me and us: We are magnificent sons and daughters of love. We are children of a living-loving-present-caring God: *Love is our nature.* We are manufactured to operate on the frequency of love. To resent,

be angry, fearful, rejecting, to criticize and blame is to stop the power and the flow of life; it is to short-circuit the frequency of love.

- The power that generates positive feelings and attitudes as well as truth, respect, support, understanding, admiration, and generosity

- The power that generates warmth, sweetness, and tenderness

- The power that generates trust, confidence, and humility

- The power that produces non-resistance, flexibility, adaptability, endurance, and the real strength of the wise

- The foundation of surrender; the power that generates self-esteem, self-worth, and self-Love. It is the power of dignity

- The Higher Power expressing in me, through me, and around me.

- My Identity/my Authentic Self

- Taking time to smell the roses, appreciate friendship, marvel, praise, and enjoy others and life

- Being able to deal with our spouse's and children's negativity; not simply tolerate it, but be at peace with it

- Being teachable, speaking the truth, saying no without feeling guilty, rendering service anonymously

**LOVE is the backbone of the program of recovery.**

## A First Step for Families

The first thing we have to do is to accept that our lives have become unmanageable. This acceptance is different from saying you cannot have control over your life. The first step is not about admitting we have a problem; it is admitting we are powerless *over* the problem. For example, when the addict returns home from treatment, we may be feeling a mixture of emotions including anxiety, concern, indecision, and fear. These emotions can cause unacceptable behaviors from us; our decision-making process is compromised and our cognitive reasoning skills become sabotaged. That is what we are powerless over; our own behaviors, not anyone else's.

The following exercise will help to understand better what "unmanageable" means and provide a clear picture of where your own life is unmanageable. This is where you have to become very honest with yourself. Later, you will have the opportunity to revisit this exercise.

## Unmanageability Exercise

Please check the following statements that apply to you

☐ Being a perfectionist

☐ Trying to control people around you

☐ Being overly defensive

☐ Being a people-pleaser

☐ Hiding behind a false self (pretending)

☐ Seeking approval from others

☐ Being a caretaker, rescuer

☐ Trying to make yourself indispensable

☐ Having little awareness of your own needs and wants

☐ Your self-worth comes from taking care of others

☐ You tell yourself "it's not that bad…"

☐ You don't know when you're tired or hungry or sick

☐ You often feel hopeless

☐ In response to your feelings and emotions, you may overeat, get sick, confused, or depressed

☐ You have difficulty trusting

☐ You have difficulty initiating things

☐ You become overly responsible

☐ You become critical and blaming

☐ You cannot express your opinions

☐ You make things up in order to please others

☐ You medicate your feelings

☐ You stay in relationships longer than you should

☐ You put up with physical or emotional abuse

☐ Your feelings may be expressed in short bombastic bursts

☐ You have difficulty identifying what you feel

☐ Your fear or anger makes you say things you normally would not

☐ You rarely talk about or share feelings

- ☐ You worry a lot
- ☐ You have difficulty making decisions
- ☐ You read about recovery rather than going into action
- ☐ You worry about someone else's problems
- ☐ You abandon your needs when you are worried
- ☐ Often you will act without thinking
- ☐ You believe you can change another person
- ☐ You want things your way
- ☐ You don't listen to your body
- ☐ You get involved with people you don't really like
- ☐ You expect others to know what you need
- ☐ You blame others because of your reality
- ☐ You feel embarrassed by the way your partner acts or dresses
- ☐ You expect others to know what you feel
- ☐ You let other people manipulate you
- ☐ You need to be the center of attention
- ☐ It's important to you that people see you as good and righteous
- ☐ Having money and possessions increase your self-worth
- ☐ You feel that your opinions are not important
- ☐ You don't say what you mean
- ☐ You yell, threaten, and blame
- ☐ You don't believe compliments given to you
- ☐ You don't like to be alone for too long
- ☐ You feel unable to change your life to be the way you want it
- ☐ You fear intimacy
- ☐ You procrastinate and put things off
- ☐ You often say things you later regret
- ☐ You get obsessed
- ☐ You don't share yourself easily
- ☐ You don't trust others

☐ You would rather not feel, so you find refuge in logic

☐ You would rather not need a relationship

☐ You sabotage your possible success

☐ You daydream about vengeance too often

☐ You get paralyzed by fear

☐ You don't feel useful or good enough

☐ You withdraw into daydreams to fulfill needs

☐ You fabricate events to bolster self-illusion

☐ You are irritated by others' assessment of you

☐ You appear lethargic and lacking vitality

☐ You become emotionally impassive or unaffectionate

☐ You become cold and humorless

☐ Your mood shifts from dejection to anger to apathy

☐ You try to keep your emotions under tight control

☐ You seem attracted to risk, danger, and harm

☐ You maintain a regulated and highly organized life

☐ You suffer from sexual preoccupation and/or acting out

☐ You become an excessive caretaker

☐ You have chronic feelings of emptiness and boredom

☐ You seek attention and praise

☐ You become competitive and power-oriented

☐ You want others to do things your way

☐ You volunteer for unpleasant tasks to gain approval

☐ You anticipate ridicule/humiliation

☐ You make suicidal attempts or threats

☐ You place yourself in inferior or demeaning positions

☐ You act arrogant and self-assured

☐ You fail to complete tasks beneficial to yourself

☐ You engage in self-sacrifice and martyrdom

☐ You feel helpless or uncomfortable when alone

- ☐ You are attracted to people who treat you poorly
- ☐ You have difficulty doing things on your own
- ☐ You tend to isolate yourself socially
- ☐ You try to control your interpersonal relationships
- ☐ You provoke rejection, then feel hurt or humiliated
- ☐ You are devastated when close relationships end
- ☐ You are fearful of loss or desertion
- ☐ You have a pattern of unstable and intense relationships
- ☐ You show little interest in sexual experiences
- ☐ You are preoccupied about the shape or appearance of your body
- ☐ You visit a physician frequently for different problems
- ☐ You often have stomach, bowel, and bladder problems
- ☐ You often have headaches, insomnia, or backaches

Were you brutally honest as you did the above exercise? Sit back for a few minutes and really do some internal soul-searching. Check within yourself to see whether you need to go back to the exercise or continue to the next process.

Now that you have acknowledged the areas that are unmanageable in your life, let's proceed to the next part of the first step process.

## Powerlessness: The First Step

Step One: "We admitted we were powerless over alcohol—that our lives had become unmanageable."

Admitting we are powerless over something means we are ready to surrender it over to our Higher Power, trusting it will be resolved in its own time. We no longer try to control the process, which has not worked for us, and only brought us frustration, unhappiness, and addictive and vicious cyclical behaviors. It is time now to admit our powerlessness and to surrender our wills and our minds over to God as we understand God.

**What are you powerless over right now?**

To Surrender is to stop and quit.
>     You STOP the Behavior/Action
>     You QUIT the Paradigm

- Surrender is giving up the outcome
- Surrender is giving up control
- Surrender is giving up old beliefs, pictures, opinions, and attitudes
- Surrender is a proactive choice that restores freedom and allows you to change your mind

**What outcomes are you still attached to or struggling with?**

**What outcomes are you trying to control?**

**Which of your old beliefs, opinions, attitudes are you giving up?**

---

**Which addictions are you giving up/stopping?**

Process Addictions (addictive behaviors)

Substance Addictions (alcohol, drugs, tobacco, food, etc.)

**What have you *really* stopped?**

---

## A Second Step for Families

Step Two: "We came to believe that a Power greater than ourselves could restore us to sanity."

Basically, the Second Step boils down to recognizing and accepting the notion of a Higher Power. It is the beginning of faith in a process and in ourselves; it is trusting that we can make changes in our lives. It may be a slow process, but when we realize that our behaviors are not unique to us—that others have made changes through their beliefs in a Higher Power—we can accept that insanity is preventing us from having a healthy relationship with the addict who has just returned home.

The concept of accepting a Higher Power may be controversial and personal, but all that is asked of you is to believe in a power greater than yourself. How you define it is really up to you, but it must be defined in an acceptable way.

You may already have your belief system in place, in which case you're already a step ahead. However, many people have never accepted a Higher Power, or have stopped believing in it. You may have tried prayer or religion, only to decide it does not work. You may have had experiences within a religion that turned you away from the idea of faith. Now you feel resistance when you are told to "come to believe." Faith may seem impossible, but trust us that it is not. You must become willing to believe in something greater than yourself, something you can turn to for help. In the beginning, it may be a support group or another person in a recovery program. At this point, your definition of Higher Power does not need to be specific; whatever you define it as, accept that a Power greater than yourself can restore you to sanity. This is what we call having a *paradigm shift* or *change of mind*.

---

**A.  What have you *really* changed your mind about?**

---

**B.  What do you really believe about...**

Yourself?


Your problem?


Your possibilities?


Your Higher Power as a solution?

C.  **Who and what do you really trust right now?**

## A Third Step for Families

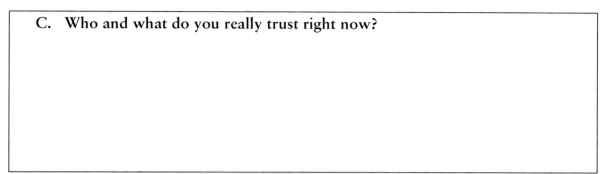

Step Three: "We made a decision to turn our will and our lives over to the care of God as we understood God."

For many people, Step Three seems impossible. You have been trying so long to control everything that it may seem beyond your ability to surrender the fear, worry, anxiety, the need to control and understand everything. This is the step where you decide to hand over your will and life to God, as you understand God.

Rest assured you are not alone. In Step One, you admitted you were powerless, which would have been difficult. But, with resources, self-confidence, self-will, self-discipline, and self-control, you were able to admit you have a problem greater than yourself, and you cannot fix it alone. And, in reality, you realized no other human being can fix it for you either. Only a Higher Power can lead you to sanity.

At this point, let's reflect a little and affirm:

God is good.

God is helping me.

Turning over your will (your thoughts) and your life (your actions) is a big step. It is about making an honest decision, but a commitment also has to be made to achieve that goal.

When you reach the Third Step, you have admitted your prior life has been out of control, and you do not have the internal peace you would like. The Third Step takes you to a place of change, a place where you are willing to be completely changed and live by the spiritual laws of creation and to be "remade" with God's guidance. It is also the place where your willingness is remade.

Now it is time to be restored to a new understanding (sanity/order.) If you feel you have made the paradigm shift and accepted that a Higher Power can restore your behaviors, complete the following exercise.

**C. What is your *new* understanding?**

How do you see *order* in your life?

Right now, what is your understanding of your Higher Power?

Intellectual Understanding (What you know.)

Feeling Understanding (What you feel.)

**D. What is your will?**

Your wants and your old ways?

Your needs and your new ways?

**E. What is your Higher Power's will for you?**

**F. What is your decision today? Will you surrender your heart and will over to God as you understand God?**

## A Fourth Step for Families

Step Four: "...Made a searching and fearless moral inventory of ourselves."

By the time our loved one seeks treatment for addiction, we have been through much frustration, outrage, embarrassment, humiliation, disappointment, and sadness. Our feelings have fluctuated between fear of what the addict might do to hurt him or herself, and our anger over our failed dreams and hope for a good life for the addict. We may also be hanging on to resentment for money we have spent to repair wrecked cars or to pay bail and medical/recovery bills.

So one of the first tasks for us is to clean the slate of these negative emotions from the past so we can move with freedom into the present. The process is simple:

Write anger letters to the addict and any other person you are angry or frustrated with. You will not mail these letters, so push all the negative emotion out of you onto the paper. Use strong language. Use a bold marker. Write in all caps. Whatever it takes to push the anger, fear, disappointment, humiliation, and outrage out of you, DO IT.

When you feel you have transferred all the raging emotion out of you onto the paper, find a safe person—a temporary Al-Anon sponsor or a trusted counselor—to read the letters to out loud. Then destroy the letters by putting them through a shredder or burning them. Now make a "searching and fearless moral inventory" of your fear and grief.

## Fear Inventory

When you experience the following fears, what is your *attitude* (i.e., compliant, defiant, dependent, submissive, angry, cynical, impulsive, jealous, etc.)? What is your *action*? What do you do? (i.e., resent, manipulate, attack, withdraw, lie, blame, get busy, procrastinate, control, etc.):

| Fear | Attitude | Action |
|------|----------|--------|
| Fear of Commitment | | |
| Fear of Intimacy | | |
| Fear of Rejection | | |
| Fear of Abandonment | | |
| Fear of Failure | | |
| Fear of Success | | |
| Fear of Change | | |
| Fear of the Unknown | | |
| Fear of Losing Control | | |
| Fear of Pain/Suffering | | |
| Fear of Being Alone | | |
| Fear of Poverty | | |
| Fear of Dying | | |

## Working with Your Fear Inventory

- Identify your fear

- Identify your attitudes and behaviors triggered by the fear

- Ask your fear what is the lesson you need to learn and the teaching that the fear is bringing. Journal the answer. If you have difficulty journaling spontaneously, use your non-dominant hand.

- Ask your fear to reveal which of your belief systems is triggering a fear response. Example: Fear of rejection—Belief is that I must be loved by everyone all the time. If I am not loved by this person, I must be bad. To be loved, I must be perfect.

- Replace your self-limiting belief with a positive one

- Remember that you are a spiritual being having a human experience

- God loves you and accepts you now

- Write an affirmation: I love myself and I accept myself fully, completely, and unconditionally

Conduct a release/cleansing ritual. It can be one of the following:

- Make a drawing of your fear and burn it. Spread the ashes outside and let the wind of freedom take it away. Then find a symbol that will represent your new belief, like a gratitude rock.

- Stand barefoot on the ground. Take a deep breath and visualize your fear or fears leaving your body through your feet. Feel the energy entering the earth. Take another breath, visualize the energy of faith entering your body through the top of your head and flowing through your entire body.

- Go for a nature walk. Find a big rock. Sit or lie on it. Feel the strength, stability, and power of the rock. Visualize yourself being part of the rock and allow strength, stability, power, and the now moment to fill every cell of your body until you feel all fear dissolved.

When your process work is done, work with an affirmation such as: I am one with God. I am faith-filled and fearless! Perfect love casts away all fear. I am grateful for my freedom.

## Stages of Grief

Following are the stages of grief as first introduced by Elisabeth Kübler-Ross in her 1969 book, *On Death and Dying*.

- **Denial:** No, it's not true. This is not happening to me.

- **Bargaining:** I'll do anything. Just change the outcome.

- **Anger:** It's not fair. You can't do that to me. How mean can you be?

- **Depression:** What's the use? The pain will never go away. I can't live like this.

- **Acceptance:** I recognize the loss and pain. I make peace with the circumstances and I see the bigger picture. I understand "why." I see my lesson. I see the gift. I experience a paradigm shift from loss to gain; from pain to a blessing.

## Grief Inventory

| |
|---|
| What are you grieving? |
| Who or what have you lost? |
| Make a list of all your losses. |
| Write a grief letter to each person or circumstance and express your feelings of loss, sadness, and grief. <br> Ask the person or circumstance to write to you and reveal to you <br> • Your lesson: <br> • Your strength and skill you have developed as a result: <br> • The blessing hidden within the pain: |

Conduct a release ritual. (It can be one of the following, or come up with your own.)

- A burning ceremony. Burn your letters.
- A burial. Make a grave and bury your pain.
- A balloon. Release a balloon to carry away your grief.
- A meaningful shower where you consciously visualize water washing away your pain.

For twenty-one days, say and write an affirmation. Examples:

- My heart is mended, my mind is healed, my feelings are cleansed, and my emotions are free.
- Love is filling every atom of my being, bringing joy, enthusiasm, and gratitude into my life. I am at peace and free.

In the Fourth Step, you identify the exact nature of your wrong. As you read these letters and inventories, could you identify times when you were judgmental? Self-righteous? Have you lied? Have you demanded perfection of an ordinary human being—either the addict or yourself? Are you overly concerned about what other people think? What has broken your heart? What was your part in the mess you have been through? *The Big Book of Alcoholics Anonymous* says:

> Putting out of our minds the wrongs others had done, we resolutely looked for our own mistakes. Where had we been selfish, dishonest, self-seeking, and frightened? Though a situation had not been entirely our fault, we tried to disregard the other person involved entirely. Where were we to blame? The inventory was ours, not the other man's. When we saw our faults, we listed them. We placed them before us in black and white. (p. 67)

To complete the Fourth Step, set an intention or say a prayer, asking that these wrongs be removed from you and transformed into something good. Here is a template to follow, a variation of the Seventh Step prayer from *The Big Book*:

> I am now willing to acknowledge that I am neither all good nor all bad, but a mixture of the two. Some of my wrongs stand in the way of healing my family relationships. I ask that they be removed and replaced with their positive opposites. Remove from me _____, _____, _____.
> Replace these negative behaviors with their positive opposites. Grant me _____, _____, and _____.

If your wrong is judgment, the positive opposite is acceptance of human nature. If your wrong is losing your temper, ask that it be replaced with peace of mind. If your wrong is perfectionism, ask for tolerance of other people's differences or your own human nature. And so on. You see how it goes. It's that simple.

If you follow this process, you will have done Steps Four, Five, Six, and Seven. Let your temporary sponsor guide you to determine whether you need to make direct amends to anyone you might have harmed or whether it would be better to make what are called "living amends." That is, change your behavior. Stop engaging in the negative and stay in the positive for longer and longer periods of time.

A Fourth Step is not a one-time process. Because we are only human, we all need a "soul cleansing" every day. Here's what *The Big Book* suggests:

> When we retire at night, we constructively review our day. Were we resentful, selfish, dishonest, or afraid? Do we owe an apology? Have we kept something to ourselves which should be discussed with another person at once? Were we kind and loving toward all? What could we have done better? Were we thinking of ourselves most of the time? Or were we thinking of what we could do for others? (p. 86)

Al-Anon is the program for family and friends of alcoholics. It was derived from Alcoholics Anonymous and also uses the Twelve Steps and Twelve Traditions, with only a few words changed. So the process laid out in *The Big Book* works for everyone in the family system of addiction.

Alcoholics and other addicts know that without the daily practice of cleansing and coming into conscious contact with a Higher Power, they might become emotionally distraught enough to drink or drug again. Families need to know that without the daily practice of cleansing and coming into conscious contact with a Higher Power, they might become emotionally drunk. That is, they might be so overcome with anger or fear that they say or do things they don't intend.

So in addition to a nightly emotional cleansing, *The Big Book* also suggests one at the beginning of every day. Following is a condensed version of pages 86-87 of *The Big Book*. We suggest that family members write these intentions every day for at least forty days:

- Today, direct my thinking.
- Divorce me from self-pity, dishonest, and self-seeking motives.
- Clear my thinking of wrong motives.
- Grant me inspiration, intuitive thought, or decision while I relax and take it easy.
- Put my thinking more and more on the plane of inspiration.

- Show me all through the day what my next step is to be and give me what I need to take it.
- Set me free from self-will. *Thy will be done.*
- Pause me through the day to ask for right thought or action.
- Discipline me with your love.

Following these morning and evening rituals, we eventually learn to "stand for ourselves but not against our fellows" (from *Survival to Recovery*). That brings us to the very important topic of communication.

## The Power of Transformation

There was a time in my life when I thought I had to
Do it all by myself...and I felt alone.

There was a time in my life when I thought I had to
Do it all...and I was overwhelmed.

There was a time in my life when I thought I had to do it
Perfectly...and I was exhausted.

There was a time in my life when I thought I had to control
People, places, moods and events...and I was frustrated.

There was a time in my life when I thought I had to know it
All...and I felt stupid and inadequate.

There was a time in my life when I thought I had to be loved
By all...and I felt rejected.

There was a time in my life when I thought I had to win and
Be right at any cost...and I felt resisted and victimized.

There was a time in my life when I thought I must avoid, kill
Or numb the pain...and I ended up stuck in my suffering.

And then there is now...
Now I release and I let go; I let my Higher Power make me whole.
Now I do the work of Steps and I let my Higher Power do the rest.

Now I am committed to putting God first in my life, knowing that God is bigger than any problem or challenge I may have. My attention is focused on the solution instead of the problem, and I am focused on my vast and mighty God.

Now I know that being happy is a choice that I make for myself right now. Regardless of appearances, I choose to be happy.

Now I allow God to take charge of my thinking and I set clear intentions with respect to the events and circumstances I desire to experience.

Now recovery is: Discovery, Transformation, Growth, Joy, and Happiness.

# 11    Changing How We Communicate

One of the definitions of the word *communicate* is "to give a share of." It is good to consider what we are giving a share of when we communicate. We have learned our communication patterns from the adults of our childhood. Thoughtlessly, we continue these patterns out of habit. But with awareness, we can discover which communication patterns do not work well for us—which ones do not allow us to "give a share of" what we truly want to share.

Gifts are provided to us when we deal with addiction in the family. One of these gifts is examining how we communicate so we can make communication choices that will enhance relationships. This is a good time to write an intention for your communication with the addict. It might go something like this: "My heart's desire is to communicate with _____ in a way that reveals my love and my belief in the highest and best within him/her."

Following is an adaptation of communication guidelines used in the Desjardins Unified Model of Treatment of Addictions:

| Roadblocks to Communication | Gate-openers for Communication |
| --- | --- |
| Moralizing, preaching: "You should..." "You ought to... It is your responsibility." | "What feels right for you?" |

Telling someone else what he or she ought to do communicates your lack of trust in that person's sense of responsibility. Over time, it cuts off communication so the person does not hear anything you have to say. On the other hand, to ask the addict, "What feels right for you?" conveys your trust in the other person and your willingness simply to be present for the current struggle or indecisiveness, with no expectations.

| Roadblocks to Communication | Gate-openers for Communication |
|---|---|
| Advising, giving solutions:<br>"What I would do is…"<br>"Why don't you…?"<br>"Let me suggest…" | "Thank you for confiding in me.<br>What do you need from me?" |

Giving unsolicited advice implies that the person is not able to solve his/her own problems. It prevents that person from thinking through a problem, considering alternative solutions, and trying them out. It can cause dependency or resistance. On the other hand, to express appreciation for candor and ask what is needed is an act of respect. With an addict, it is essential to establish your boundaries before you ask this question. Then, if the addict asks for something that violates your boundary, you can say, "No, I can't do that. But I can do this."

| Roadblocks to Communication | Gate-openers for Communication |
|---|---|
| Judging, criticizing, blaming:<br>"You are not thinking maturely."<br>"You are lazy." | Be silent. Or say how you're feeling. |

When we criticize someone, we run the risk of cutting off communication altogether; no one wants to be "bawled out." It invites defensiveness and counter-attack. In your silence, it's good to be saying the Serenity Prayer internally. Or silently ask God to do for you what you cannot do. Or ask God to give you the words that are needed. Then, when you are completely calm, speak from your heart. If you are feeling angry, disappointed, or afraid, *remain silent*. Or say, "I'm feeling afraid for you"—and leave it at that.

| Roadblocks to Communication | Gate-openers for Communication |
|---|---|
| **Diversion:** "Let's talk about something pleasant."<br>**Sarcasm:** Why don't you try running the World?"<br>**Withdrawal:** (Giving the silent treatment) | "This is difficult for me to hear, but I'm willing to listen."<br>"I don't have anything to say, but I want you to know I heard every word."<br>"I don't like what you're saying, but I love you." |

Relationships are damaged by diverting, being sarcastic, and withdrawing. All of these behaviors are forms of rejection. A challenging aspect of recovery is accepting what we do not like, yet cannot change. Our communication must reflect this acceptance.

| Roadblocks to Communication | Gate-openers for Communication |
|---|---|
| Ordering, commanding:<br>"You must..."<br>"You have to..."<br>"You will..." | "Make the decision that's right for you." |

Commands invite active resistance, "testing." They promote rebellious behavior and retaliation. An Al-Anon slogan encourages people to "stand for ourselves but not against our fellows." In other words, say what you want with the realization that you have no power whatsoever over what the other person does.

| Roadblocks to Communication | Gate-openers for Communication |
|---|---|
| Warning, threatening:<br>"If you don't, then..."<br>"You'd better, or...". | Say what you mean, mean what you say, and do what you say. |

Threatening can produce fear or submissiveness, as well as invite "testing" of the consequences you threatened. It can actually cause resentment, anger, and rebellion. On the other hand, from a calm state of mind, get clear on what you truly need to say. Once you've said it, follow through immediately.

| Roadblocks to Communication | Gate-openers for Communication |
|---|---|
| Unmerited praise or agreement:<br>"You're doing a great job, no matter what your boss says...<br>You're right!<br>That teacher sounds awful!<br>That cop must have needed to make a quota." | Acknowledge that we're all only human, and we can learn from our mistakes.<br>We don't have to be perfect to be loved |

Sometimes referred to as "taking someone's side," the comments on the left imply that the loved one has to be right in order to be accepted. Such comments actually create anxiety and disconnect the person from truth and the opportunity to learn. On the other hand, facing the truth with someone and having confidence that he or she will learn from the experience is truly an act of love.

| Roadblocks to Communication | Gate-openers for Communication |
|---|---|
| Probing, questioning: "Why? Who? How?" | Listen to understand. |

Interrogation invites resistance and cover-up. People tend to reply with non-answers, avoidance, half-truths, or lies. The focus shifts from telling the truth to placating the questioner so he or she will stop. The preferable alternative is to listen without interruption until the speaker has told the whole story. Make it comfortable for him or her to tell the truth.

| Roadblocks to Communication | Gate-openers for Communication |
|---|---|
| Name-calling, ridiculing: "Crybaby..." "Okay, Mr. Smarty..." | No ridicule. *Ever.* Listen and speak affirmatively. |

Name-calling and ridiculing will strip people of their dignity. Such talk can cause the person to feel unworthy and unloved. It has a devastating effect on self-image and often provokes verbal and even physical retaliation. An old African-American expression is, "He called me out of my name." That's a very good description of what actually happens in our hearts and minds when someone does this.

| Roadblocks to Communication | Gate-openers for Communication |
|---|---|
| Correcting, instructing: "You should do it this way..." "You did it wrong..." "You made a mistake." | Ask yourself: "How important is. it?" "Would you rather be right, or would you rather be happy?" |

When my son was a teenager, he once worked outside, all day digging postholes, setting posts, and stringing barbed wire for our pasture fence. He made a decision upon beginning to let the fence follow the undulations of the land. But when his father got home, he didn't like the unevenness of the lines. He showed no appreciation for his son's effort and immediately began explaining what was wrong and how it had to be corrected. He even got out his level tool to prove his point. That was over twenty years ago, and my son still has not forgotten or forgiven his father for his harsh, self-righteous words, with no acknowledgement or appreciation for the effort he had made.

| Roadblocks to Communication | Gate-openers for Communication |
|---|---|
| Complaining, self-disclosing, and self-pity:<br>"Poor me!"<br>"I have so many problems…"<br>Did I tell you about my operation…?<br>"No one can help me now." | Ask about the other person. Show interest in him or her.<br>Talking about your problems intensifies them.<br>Let your conversation be uplifting. |

People avoid those who complain too much. It's impossible to engage someone in a meaningful, two-way conversation when it is so closely focused on one person's problems. The conversation leads nowhere. The listener feels used and resents the self-centered approach.

Once I had a friend who was anticipating major back surgery. I was willing to listen to her, up to a point, but once the decision was made to have the surgery, there was no point in continuing to go over and over the problem that was about to be corrected. One day, when I met her for coffee, she brought her x-rays for me to see. When she pulled them out, I simply said, "I do not want to see your x-rays. I just want to enjoy some idle conversation with you. Have you seen any good movies lately?" She laughed, and we changed the subject.

| Roadblocks to Communication | Gate-openers for Communication |
|---|---|
| Analyzing, diagnosing:<br>"What's wrong with you is…"<br>"You're just tired…"<br>"You don't really mean that." | It's not your job to analyze other people; it's your job to appreciate them and just hear them out without injecting your opinion |

The comments on the left are conversation-stoppers. They level judgment and create an unsafe climate for meaningful conversation. The alternative is just to listen, or simply to say, "I hear you."

| Roadblocks to Communication | Gate-openers for Communication |
|---|---|
| Persuading with logic, arguing—<br>"Here's why you are wrong…"<br>"The facts are…"<br>"Yes, but…" | Listen with appreciation to opinions different from yours.<br>Ask questions for clarification, with the intent of understanding. |

Arguing is so tiresome. People become passionate; they interrupt each other; they try to prove themselves right and everyone else wrong. People quit listening and become defensive.

Instead, from a quiet state of mind, ask questions for clarification. Your intention is only to understand. The opportunity for learning and shared meaning will increase greatly.

| Roadblocks to Communication | Gate-openers for Communication |
|---|---|
| Reassuring, sympathizing:<br>"Don't worry…"<br>"You'll feel better tomorrow…"<br>"Oh, cheer up." | "I'm so sorry that happened to you." |

Empathize. Don't minimize. Don't gloss over or try to convince someone it's not important. Empathize.

# 12 Understanding Codependent Roles

Addictions affect each member of the family, from the unborn child to the addict's spouse, partner, parents, and siblings. The addiction results not only in physical problems for the addict, but also in physical and psychological problems for family members. In most cases, treatment is complicated, and often not completely successful without a total understanding of codependency. Even if the addict eventually abstains, the family members may never recover from the problems inflicted upon them.

Codependency is not recognized as a diagnosable disorder, according to the American Psychiatric Association's *Diagnostic and Statistical Manual of Mental Disorders*. However, codependence, according to the National Council on Codependence, refers to the present effect of events from our childhood on our attitude, thoughts, and behaviors. The Council defines codependency as:

> A learned behavior, expressed by dependencies on people and things outside the self: these dependencies include neglecting and diminishing of one's own identity. The false self that emerges is often expressed through compulsive habits, addictions, and other disorders that further increase alienation from the person's true identity, fostering a sense of shame. (1990)

Codependency is a maladaptive bonding with a family system. To survive psychologically and socially in this dysfunctional family, the child adopts patterns of thinking, acting, and feeling that, at first, dull the pain, but finally are self-negating in themselves. These patterns may become:

Caretaker ~ People Pleaser ~ Martyr

Compulsive Performer ~ Perfectionist ~ Tap Dancer

These effects are potentially destructive because codependency is an unconscious addiction to another person's abnormal behavior. When the addict goes through a recovery process, he or she seemingly does well, leading the codependent person to believe the problem has been solved. Often, codependent family members do everything possible to hide the problem or indicate that the addict is no longer an addict, thus attempting to preserve the family's reputation.

Concentrating on projecting an image of a "perfect family," codependent family members often forget about their own needs and desires. They dedicate their lives to attempting to control or to prevent the addict from relapsing. Unknowingly, codependent family members often become "enablers." An enabler is a person who unknowingly denies that a problem exists, rescues the addict from destructive behaviors, makes excuses, or lies. Any time a family member allows the addict to continue in unproductive/addictive behavior, whether actively or passively, enabling occurs. Often, if the family says nothing, it is also an enabling behavior; it gives the addict silent permission to continue the same behavior. Silence is often caused by fear—fear of hurting the addict; fear of retaliation; fear of the addict hurting, hating, or not liking you; fear of being hit or worse; fear of butting in where you don't think you belong.

Before we define the typical characteristics of codependency, we ask you to re-visit the statements you checked under the manageability exercise (p. 77).

# Typical Characteristics of Codependency

☐ You assume responsibility for the addict's feelings and/or behaviors.

☐ You feel overly responsible for the addict or other family members' feelings and/or behaviors.

☐ You have difficulty identifying or expressing feelings. *Am I angry? Lonely? Sad? Happy? Joyful?*

☐ You fear and/or worry how others, particularly the addict, will respond to your feelings.

☐ You are afraid of being hurt and/or rejected by the addict and other family members.

☐ You have difficulty in forming and/or maintaining close relationships.

☐ You are afraid of being hurt and/or rejected by others.

☐ You are a perfectionist and place expectations on yourself, the addict, and other family members.

☐ You have difficulty making the "right" decision, or any decision.

☐ You minimize, alter, or deny the truth of your feelings.

☐ Your fear of others' feelings (anger) determines what you say or do.

☐ Your responses, actions, and reactions are determined by other people's actions and attitudes.

☐ You put other people's needs and wants before your own.

☐ Your self-esteem is bolstered by outer/other influences. You cannot acknowledge good things about yourself.

☐ You question or ignore your own values and tend to value others' opinions.

☐ You cannot acknowledge good things about yourself and your self-esteem is strengthened by outer influences.

☐ Your serenity and mental attention are determined by how others are feeling and or behaving.

Each family member may be affected by the addict's behavior differently, usually dependent on that person's degree of codependency. Codependency is a behavioral pattern that deprives individuals of their hopes, dreams, desires, and even needs. Codependents allow others' behaviors and addictions to influence and dictate their lives. Recognizing codependent behavior is the first step in overcoming it and regaining control of our own lives, rather than focusing on the addict's behavior.

## Codependent Profile

A codependent person may have all or some of these conditions.

| Physically | Emotionally |
|---|---|
| • Drained/Tired | • Insecure |
| • Depressed | • Fearful |
| • Restless Sleep | • Worried |
| • Digestive Problems | • Anxious |
| • Headaches | • Guilty |
| • Backaches | • Frustrated |
| • Asthma/Allergies | • Angry |
| • Eating Disorders | • Resentful |
| • PMS Problems | • Numb |
| • Sexual Anorexia or Dysfunction | |

| Mentally | Effects |
|---|---|
| • Preoccupied | • People Pleasing |
| • Scattered | • Approval Seeking |
| • Overwhelmed | • Needy |
| • Controlling | • Dependent |
| • Rigid | • Immature |
| • Questioning/Probing | • Fixer and Martyr |
| • Self-Centered | |
| • Issue-Oriented and Problem Oriented | |
| • Seeing the Small Picture and Symptoms | |
| • Obsessive/Compulsive | |

Being a codependent isn't easy. It requires a lot of work and it hurts. If you recognize any of the behaviors in the list below, you know how difficult it is. While you may be critical of your own dysfunctional behavior, you are also very good at justifying the dysfunctional behavior of others.

## Codependent Behaviors

- Messiah Complex
- Fixer
- Enabler
- Drama Queen or King
- Caretaker vs. Caregiver
- Saintly Martyr
- Need to be Indispensable
- Feed Off Other People's Problems

Codependents are approval-driven and allow themselves to be affected if others are angry at them or disappointed with them. As such, they place themselves in roles of Caretaker, People Pleaser, Workaholic, Martyr, Perfectionist and/or Tap Dancer. It is possible that a codependent may play all these roles, some more strongly than the others.

Following is the description of each role you may play, and an assignment to help determine how your roles affect your relationships.

# Codependent Roles

## Caretaker

| Behaviors |
|---|
| Fixing ~ Lecturing ~ Correcting ~ Probing ~ Rescuing ~ Protecting ~ Lying<br>Minimizing ~ Smothering ~ Clinging ~ Possessing ~ Depending ~ Controlling |
| **Assignment :** Write how your caretaking affects the following: |
| Family Relationships (primary) |
| Work Related Relationships |
| Social Relationships |
| Rate this behavior on a scale of 1 - 10 (10 = Most problematic) _____ |

## People Pleaser

| Behaviors |
|---|
| Suppressing Feelings and Needs ~ Dishonest Talk ~ Assuming ~ Minimizing<br>Exaggerating ~ Manipulating ~ Controlling ~ Avoiding |
| **Assignment:** Write how your people pleasing affects the following: |
| Family Relationships (primary) |
| Work Related Relationships |
| Social Relationships |
| Rate this behavior on a scale of 1 - 10 (10 = Most problematic) _____ |

## Workaholic

| Behaviors |
|---|
| Overachieving ~ Pressurizing ~ Demanding ~ Creating Chaos<br>Procrastinating/Blaming ~ Getting Validated ~ Escaping ~ Controlling |
| **Assignment:** Write how your workaholic behavior affects the following: |
| Family Relationships (primary) |
| Work Related Relationships |
| Social Relationships |
| Rate this behavior on a scale of 1 - 10 (10 = Most problematic) _____ |

**Martyr**

| **Behaviors** |
|---|
| Guilt Tripping Others ~ Self Sacrificing ~ Enabling Actions |
| Suffering ~ Depression ~ Controlling with Pain/Illness |

| **Assignment:** Write how your martyr behavior affects the following: |
|---|
| Family Relationships (primary) |
| Work Related Relationships |
| Social Relationships |
| Rate this behavior on a scale of 1 - 10 (10 = Most problematic) _____ |

## Perfectionist

| Behaviors |
| --- |
| Setting Unrealistic Goals and Expectations ~ Setting Rigid and Unrealistic Boundaries ~Competing ~ Comparing ~ Criticizing ~ Humiliating ~ Rigid Uncompromising Thinking and Feeling |

**Assignment:** Write how your perfectionism affects the following:

Family Relationships (primary)

Work Related Relationships

Social Relationships

Rate this behavior on a scale of 1 - 10 (10 = Most problematic) _____

## Tap Dancer

| Behaviors |
|---|
| Avoiding Commitment ~ Giving Double Messages ~ Triangular Talk |
| Aloof ~ Making False Promises ~ Confusing ~ Distant ~ Secretive |
| Enticing ~ Alluring ~ Moody ~ Resistant ~ Inconsistent ~ Unrealistic |

**Assignment:** Write how your tap dancing behavior affects the following:

Family Relationships (primary)




Work Related Relationships




Social Relationships




Rate this behavior on a scale of 1 - 10 (10 = Most problematic) _____

A healthy relationship with the addict or other family member is based on interdependence. Codependence and interdependence are two very different dynamics. Codependence is giving away our power. Interdependence is forming partnerships, alliances and connections with others.

Taking our self-definition and self-worth from external sources is dysfunctional because it causes us to give power over our feelings about ourselves to people and forces we cannot control. The way to healthy interdependence is to see things clearly—to see people, situations, life dynamics, and most of all ourselves, clearly. If we are not working on healing our wounds and changing our programming, we cannot have a clear view of ourselves or anything else that goes on in our lives.

## Behavioral Patterns of Codependency and Interdependency

| Codependency | Interdependency |
| --- | --- |
| Caretaker | Helper |
| People Pleaser | Communicator |
| Workaholic | Peak Performer |
| Martyr | Enthusiast |
| Perfectionist | Possibility Thinker |
| Tap Dancer | Artist/Co-Creator |

By changing our paradigm—attitudes, beliefs, and definitions—we can stop expecting life to be something it is not. Unless we start having a realistic view of our relationships, we can stop expecting our relationship with the addict, or other family members, to do well. A realistic view will allow us to be responsible enough to work through issues, to keep communication happening, to form a healthy interdependent partnership with another human being. By taking responsibility and working through issues, we can experience acceptance of the addict and of ourselves.

# 13 Understanding Our Own Codependency

Before we can accept or support the addict, we need to look at our own codependency. We must acknowledge that codependency is not healthy, and if an addiction in another person is identified, we have to reassess and make changes in our lives. This same acknowledgement will require us to be honest with ourselves; we often cannot grasp the concept of honesty because essentially it opposes addiction. Addiction is running away from the self; it is fear, dishonesty, disloyalty, untrustworthiness, and falseness. It is not knowing how to love the self because loving the self is self-acceptance; when we fear facing the truth of our feelings, we do not accept ourselves.

Our codependency may become the ego's key motivating force. We attempt to fill our being with something outside ourselves, becoming disconnected from the love within us. Through codependency, we hide from self-judgment and hatred, as well as shame and guilt we don't want to face. The result comes in addiction to substances (alcohol, drugs, nicotine), or it may show up as workaholism, relationship addiction, overeating, or even caring for others. Essentially, anything that takes us away from our own feelings is codependency.

Outside conflicts and inner pressures may trigger any one of these results at any time. Understanding codependency helps to understand the addict and why he or she chose to resort to substances. However, it also gives us the knowledge that we, as family members or friends of the addict, need to assess our own codependency and how we respond to him or her. We have to be extremely careful that our own behaviors and feelings do not convert into codependency, thereby damaging both the relationship with the addict and with ourselves.

It's not easy. Regardless of possible negative consequences, our better judgment is often overwhelmed and we continually choose the object of our own behavior. We give our power away to our addictive behaviors rather than to what serves our highest good. Consequently, the shame, regret, and judgment of betraying ourselves pave the way to guilt, self-criticism, and remorse. Of course, a very fitting part of addiction is that we ardently deny that any pain or suffering we experience in our lives has anything to do with our own behaviors. Most often, the ones closest to us take blame for the chaos our behavior generates. Instead, we must acknowledge our powerlessness over the addict, acknowledge that our codependent behavior can harm us, and take responsibility for making changes in our own lives before we can support the addict.

This perspective may be different from what you have read or heard about and may be different from what the addict learned in the treatment center. We will not enter into a debate of what is right or wrong; we simply take it a level deeper by acknowledging that the truth is within us. The first step in healing our own behaviors is to acknowledge that we have abandoned ourselves. The reasons for abandonment are many and they are not important at this point. What is important is getting rid of the constant judging, criticism, and labeling that come to us through our internal dialogue. If the noise of the rejected behavior, the old patterns or tapes playing in our heads, is overwhelming, then work on the self must become a priority over understanding and supporting the addict. Our willingness to take responsibility for our lives may be the best healing process the recovering addict can experience. By surrendering our own behaviors and releasing old wounds we can become fully present and set an example for the addict to follow.

> "Fear is the tax which conscience pays to guilt."
> ~ Author Unknown

# 14 Coping Skills

These skills are composed of four ingredients:

**1. Patience:**

- Peaceful anticipation
- True and treasured insights
- Empowering new creative energy
- Without patience, we are stuck in an addictive mode of:
    - Impulsivity
    - Crisis Creating, dramas, projections
    - Core Addictions and Ego reactions

**2. De-dramatization of Reality:**

- Ability to see the big picture beyond appearances
- willingness to understand before being understood
- Flexibility and openness of mind
- Ability to laugh at oneself

**3. Surrender:**

- Ability to give up attachments to outcomes
- Ability to trust a Higher Power and believe in Divine Order
- Ability to make proactive choices = Giving up the need to being right and choosing to be happy and in harmony

**4. Acceptance:**

- Giving up the belief in and the need for struggle
- Embracing what is vs. being stuck in wishful thinking

When situations we don't like arise, or when someone behaves in a manner that offends us, we tend to react. Our reactivity is lightning-fast; we experience, in the words of Joseph LeDoux, "emotional hijackings," and we end up in a state of mind that we don't like. We don't even realize that we had a choice in the matter and that we chose to go along with the hijacking. To move from coping with the family disease of alcoholism to transforming our lives requires awareness that we have a choice.

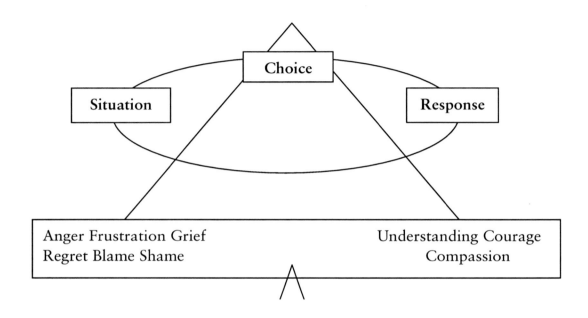

Recovery requires interrupting the cycle of situation/response that throws us into negativity. All of us have an inner "dial" that can disengage from the emotion of the moment and choose a state of mind that is likely to bring about healing and reconciliation. This is a process of "emotional sobriety" that ideally all family members, including the addict, acquire, slowly and steadily, over time.

Moving from negativity into more desirable states of mind isn't usually done quickly, like flipping a switch. Most people, however, can move from negativity into neutrality—withholding judgment, for example; or simply understanding. In a program developed for family members, a dramatization depicted the addict with a second person holding a hand puppet over one shoulder of the addict, to demonstrate that there is a disease that has a life of its own, and family members have to learn to distinguish who is speaking—the addict or the disease. This understanding helps to dislodge negativity's hold.

The work of David Hawkins indicates that courage opens the door to neutrality. "Courage" is derived from the French word for heart—*coeur*. It's getting out of one's head, trying to figure out what to do and how to do it to get the desired results. It's moving into our hearts, asking what Love would do.

Many of us spend so much time in our heads that we don't even know how to listen to our hearts. For these people, the following process helps:

1. Put your hand over your heart. Close your eyes. Take four long, deep breaths—all the way from your navel. Slowly count to four on the inhale and four on the exhale.

2. Feel the warmth from your hand penetrating your skin and even going into your heart. Now feel your heart beating. Realize that this heart started beating in the third week after your conception, and it will continue to beat until your very last breath, faithfully pumping, replenishing, and refreshing your body—sustaining your life. Thank your heart for its faithfulness in sustaining your life.

3. Ask your heart what to do in this current situation. Just ask the question and just sit with the question. If your head tries to answer, ignore it. The heart's message is often silent—it's an inner knowing.

4. For a few minutes, just sit, breathing deeply and regularly.

5. Take one final long, deep breath—all the way from your navel. Slowly open your eyes, put your hand down, and feel the peace. Realize that courage comes from the heart. Now rewrite your script with courage.

# Part III:

# Rewriting The Script

Love unconditionally,
everything that was once difficult
will become easy.

Love unconditionally,
everything that was once complicated
will become simple.

Love unconditionally,
everything that was once broken
will become whole.

Philip M. Berk
*Mountain's Stillness, River's Wisdom:*
*A Compassionate Guide to the Art of Being*

| 15 | # Moving Forward<br># To Rewrite The Script |
|---|---|

Perhaps the greatest surprise of having a loved one go into recovery is the realization that it is we ourselves who must change. We must "rewrite the script" we are living. To paraphrase Gandhi, "We must become the change we want to see [in the alcoholic/addict]." The destination of this transformation is unconditional love.

The process may be likened to the metamorphosis a caterpillar makes in becoming a butterfly, described by Anodea Judith in *Waking the Global Heart* (p. 36):

> Within the chrysalis a miracle occurs. Tiny cells, called "maginal cells," begin to appear. These cells are wholly different from caterpillar cells, carrying different information, vibrating to a different frequency—the frequency of the emerging butterfly. At first, the caterpillar's immune system perceives these new cells as enemies and attacks them, much as new ideas are called radical, and viciously denounced by the powers now holding center stage. But the maginal cells are not deterred. They continue to appear, increasing in numbers until the new cells are numerous enough to organize into clumps. When enough cells have formed to make structures along the *new* organizational lines, the caterpillar's immune system is overwhelmed. The cells of the original body then become a nutritious soup for the growth of the butterfly.

Similarly, it's common for a family struggling with someone's addiction to be outraged and attack the idea that they might own part of the problem. They think if the addict would quit using and just behave him or herself, everything would be fine. They reject the idea of change for themselves. The transformational process is gradual, incremental, and often uncomfortable. It's an organic process, constantly evolving. That's why it is taken *one step at a time*.

Gilles and Liliane Desjardins have been working with this process for over thirty years. They are renowned for their highly successful and innovative work with the Desjardins Unified Model of Treatment of Addictions.

The Desjardins' process works for all addictions, including codependency. According to Liliane Desjardins, "15% of addiction has to do with a chemical; the other 85% is state of mind issues."

The point of reference for the necessary transformation is from living out of the ego/personality to living out of the identity/authentic self.

The following chart was created by the Desjardins' to illustrate this shift.

| Ego/Personality | Identity/Authentic Self |
|---|---|
| **Negative Self:** | **Positive Self:** |
| • Negative beliefs and imprints | • Positive beliefs and imprints |
| • Negative self-perception | • Positive self-perceptions |
| • Negative self-esteem | • Positive self-esteem |
| • Negative self-image and self-worth | • Positive self-image and self-worth |
| **Negative and/or addictive:** | **Positive and empowering:** |
| • Attitudes | • Attitudes |
| • Behaviors | • Behaviors |
| • Self-limiting and self-destructive patterns | • Creative, constructive habits and patterns |
| • Character defects | • Strengths, talents, and skills |
| **Sees self as a human being trying to have a spiritual experience** | **Sees self as a spiritual being having many human experiences** |
| Ego is the condition developed when the personality grows disproportionately larger in comparison to identity/authentic self. | Identity/authentic self is aligned with universal principles, the self that is in the image and likeness of God. |
| It is a state engendered by chronic denial, which is rooted in the unrealistic notion of control. | Identity is the spiritual self: positive, constructive, freeing, and creative. |
| Control is at the core of addictions. It is an obsessive need to oversee every detail in all aspects of one's life and affairs. Coupled with this obsession is the perception that others are an extension of self and therefore within one's right to dominate. | Identity is our spiritual DNA, connected to spiritual and natural laws and principles of growth, maturity, love, wisdom, strength, integrity. |
| Control is the addictive link between the addict and the co-addict. | |

Surrender is the first phase of this shift.

## What Is Surrender?

Surrender is:

- To realize the futility of repeating the same patterns and expecting different results.

- To realize the pain and struggle caused by trying to control outcomes.

- Being in the now.

- The desire for change and something better.

- The realization that I don't know and I don't have the answer.

- The realization that I need help.

- The willingness to ask for help.

- The willingness to let go of outcomes.

- The willingness and humility to experience my vulnerability.

- The beginning of trust.


Surrender Is Embracing:

- Our Identity

- Our Authentic Self

- The Excellence Within

## How Does Surrender Manifest?

| | |
|---|---|
| **Physical Level** | I am present.<br>I breathe in and out.<br>I take a deep breath. I exhale slowly.<br>I become aware of my body.<br>I relax my body; I let go of the tenseness in all my joints and muscles. |
| **Intellectual Level** | I am in the now.<br>I am aware of my thoughts.<br>I stop the inner chatter and struggle.<br>I stop the resistance and denial.<br>I stop the delusional thoughts.<br>I focus on letting go.<br>I become aware of what goes on in my mind.<br>I consciously choose not to give power to the negative thoughts.<br>I use my breath and an affirmation: I breathe in peace and release; I breathe out tension and struggle |
| **Emotional Level** | I am here, present in the now.<br>I listen and let my breath open up my heart and lungs.<br>I feel vulnerable but safe.<br>I feel tired and exhausted from the fight.<br>I feel powerless to solve my problems.<br>I feel fearful of the unknown but hopeful. |
| **Spiritual Level** | Through my breath, I reconnect with my body, mind, emotions, and spirit.<br>I am connected, and I believe that of myself, I cannot do it.<br>I do come to believe that I need the help of a power greater than me—God or a Higher Power. |

My fear and mistrust level are lowered and are replaced with hope and trust.

I experience paradoxical thinking/feeling:

As I admit my powerlessness over my negative imprints/perceptions, feelings, attitudes, and behaviors, I become *empowered.*

*I EXPERIENCE A PARADIGM SHIFT = A SHIFT IN MY BELIEF SYSTEM*

## After Surrender Comes Forgiveness

Following is the Desjardins' process for forgiveness, beginning with understanding the causes of not forgiving and subsequent responses, causes, and consequences of anger and resentment, and finally, a process for setting ourselves free by forgiving all of it.

## The Process of Unforgiveness

Causes: Injustice—Victimization—Betrayal—Disempowerment
             Violence—Losses—Our Perceptions—Our Perfectionism

Our False Pride and Self-Righteousness

Responses: Fear—Shame—Guilt—Anger—Blame—Resentment—Hate

When we justify our resentments because we feel we "have a right to feel this way," it is like drinking a cup of poison and expecting someone else to die.

## Anger Has Many Faces

Anger is:

- A fear-based response to perceived danger, injustice, or opposition.
- Broadly applied to feelings of resentful or vengeful displeasure.
- A power and control tool used as self-defense or for attack.
- A drain of positive energy.

Anger has different intensities. It goes from irritation...to resentments...to rage...to fury...to madness.

Anger, if self-directed and unaddressed, can lead to suicide. If other-directed and unaddressed, anger can lead to homicide.

Anger can be suppressed and then manifested in passive resistance.

Anger can be expressed as criticism, blame, and verbal abuse, or as silent rejection or neglect and emotional abuse.

Anger can be violently expressed as rage and/or physical, sexual, financial, and/or religious abuse.

## Resentment Triggers That Keep Us Stuck In Unforgiveness

- Our addiction to security, power/control, sensation, and suffering
- Other people's expectations
- Loss of self
- Deprivation/Abandonment
- Abuse
- Envy
- Worry
- Perfectionism
- False Pride
- Self-righteousness
- Unfinished business/Lack of closure
- Over commitment
- Holding on to loss

## Steps of Forgiveness

- Confront your emotional pain, your shock, fear, anger, and grief.
- Recognize that the hurt that has occurred may have been unfair and that these steps are not meant to minimize the hurt involved.
- Realize that forgiveness can only be appropriate after you have processed your fear, anger, and grief.
- Understand that LOVE is what you ultimately want for you from you, and forgiveness is a gift you are giving yourself by reclaiming your power.
- Understand that forgiveness does not condone, approve, or forget the harmful acts.
- Realize that you are the only person capable of and responsible for your own feelings and for healing the hurt inside you. Forgiveness can happen only in the NOW moment.

| 16 | **Transformation and The Twelve Steps** |
|---|---|

(Used with permission from Gilles and Liliane Desjardins)

The Twelve Steps provide the foundation of our transformation. It all begins and ends with these simple steps, which will keep us on the path that leads to self-actualization, love, and success.

Recovery/Transformation is a spiritual process of re-creating our lives. As with all spiritual things, the process is composed of paradoxes:

- When we admit powerlessness, we become empowered.

- When we admit loss of control, we start experiencing manageability of our affairs.

- When we admit defeat, we begin winning.

- When we ask for help, we are no more isolated.

- When we start a new *belief system* and set a new *intention*, our entire biochemistry responds, and we align ourselves with the Universal Energy that sustains us.

The Steps, when practiced, turn these paradoxes into reality. Through the practice of these Steps, self-rejection and self-hatred are transformed into love of self, love of God, and love of others. Failures turn into success, and life has a deeper meaning.

The twelve steps are a foolproof system
For the life that we seek, need, and want!

## Priorities and the Twelve Steps

As addiction in families strengthens over time, priorities slip. In many cases, getting the addict sober becomes an all-consuming focus, leaving other family members without attention and even neglecting themselves in pursuit of sobriety for someone else. So the Twelve Steps re-prioritize our relationships. Simply stated, it's God first, ourselves second, and everything else somewhere further down the line. The Desjardins developed the following two charts to illustrate:

### Relationships—Order of Priorities

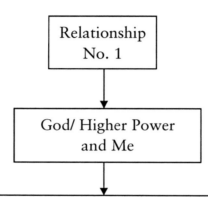

Relationship
No. 1

God/ Higher Power
and Me

**My Understanding Of God/Higher Power**

God = in the now vs. past or future

God = acting now in me and through me vs. a deity "out there"

God = healing energy of love vs. frightening, punitive Judge

God = expressed through identity

God = my perfect parent—perfect love

God = power present and acting when I am powerless and surrendered

My time and my attention and my focus must be given to this relationship that keeps me connected to my identity vs. my ego.

I must grow in my spiritual awareness, which is the basis for my maturity.

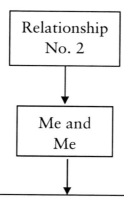

**My Understanding of Me**

I am a recovering _____.

I am a child of God; I am OK.

I am loving and lovable.

I have a purpose: to be and express my identity.

I love myself.

I appreciate myself.

I approve of myself.

I am worthy.

I am enough.

I respect myself.

I enjoy my company.

I am nice to be with.

My time and attention and my focus must be given to this relationship that gives me balance between my divine and my human self.

I can give to the others only who and what I am.

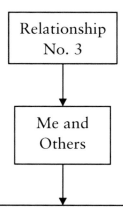

**My relationship with significant others**
a.  Spouse/lover/girlfriend/boyfriend
b.  Children
c.  Parents
d.  Working relationships
e.  Friends
f.  Society/community

**Who I am in each of these roles.**

I fulfill these roles, but I do not identify with them: I am more than that.

I bring the best of me into each as they are not my false gods.

**The Twelve Steps and Relationships**

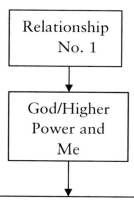

Relationship
No. 1

God/Higher
Power and
Me

STEPS TO USE:
<u>FIRST STEP</u>:  Admit powerlessness, ask for help.
<u>SECOND STEP</u>:  We came to believe…
    Higher Power can restore us to sanity = divine
order.
<u>THIRD STEP</u>:  Decision and understanding.
    We turn our will and our lives over to the care
of a Higher Power.

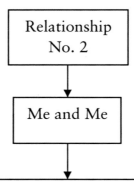

Relationship
No. 2

Me and Me

STEPS TO USE:

FOURTH STEP:  Fearless inventory of my diseased ego and self-discovery of my behavior.

FIFTH STEP:  Admission of my wrongs to God, self, and others = out of denial, reconnected out of isolation and dry drunk.

SIXTH STEP:  I fully consent to give up my ego and my goofiness—God change me at depth. I take responsibility for my life.

SEVENTH STEP:  Humility = I can't do it alone; I need God's help. God removes my negativity. I concentrate and go into action by using my twelve powers and my twelve strengths; I let my identity flow.

TENTH STEP:  I keep growing daily by processing the "ego attacks." The Tenth Step is the tool to keep me out of addiction in my free power of choice. It is prevention for being a good dry drunk.

ELEVENTH STEP:  Through prayer and meditation, we establish a conscious contact with God = with higher self/with our life and our purpose.

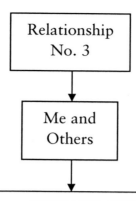

STEPS TO USE:

<u>EIGHTH STEP</u>: A list of people I have hurt (in the past). Mainly a list of who I am hurting now and to whom I need to make amends.

<u>NINTH STEP</u>: I make my amends to people I hurt.
  I repair the damage.
  I change my attitudes and behavior.
  I quit letting my ego ruin my life and my relationships.

<u>TWELFTH STEP</u>:
  My spiritual awakening has taken place.
  I do not react out of ego. I act out of identity.
  I carry the message of my transformation into my relationships.
  My actions and my <u>being</u> speak louder than any word I can say.
  I practice the principles in my relationships with others = honesty, humility—hope—purity of intent—and love.

"We serve others when we do what is right for ourselves."
—Author Unknown

# 17   Practicing the Principle of Love

Most of us have heard the adage, "Charity begins at home." Unfortunately, most people believe love is something that comes to us from outside ourselves—something we give or get. But practicing the principle of love means loving ourselves and thereby becoming equipped to give it to others. Liliane Desjardins says, "Many people don't know how to love. They know how to rescue, how to advise, how to try to improve others, how to provide with material possessions. But they don't know how to love. Love begins with self-love."

## What is self-love?

Self-love is:
A deep sense of self-worth.
An ennobling sense of self-respect.
A divine awareness of personal dignity.
A sincere belief in myself.
Self-love is:
Knowing I am wanted ⎫
Knowing I am needed ⎬ by God / by Me / by Others
Knowing I am trusted ⎭
Knowing I am present and connected.
Knowing I am:  Dependable
                  Reliable
                  Consistent
                  Responsible
                  Generous
                  Understanding
                  Patient
                  Kind

## Forgiving

Self-love is

- Knowing I make a difference.
- Giving my love to someone who needs me.
- Being true to my highest ideals.
- Respecting and fulfilling my deepest needs and not giving in to my addictive, immature wants.
- Respecting, listening to, and following my intuition.
- Coming, being, and acting out of my identity instead of my ego.
- Going for my highest goals.
- Having a personal code of ethics enhancing self and others.

Self-love is

- Being proud of myself.
- Being happy with myself.
- Being proud of my country and my origins.
- Living beyond humiliation and embarrassment.
- Living beyond racial, cultural, or religious prejudices.
- Living beyond what I believe my human limitations are.

Self-love is

- Being honest—the incredible feeling of freedom that honesty gives me.
- Being real and genuine.
- Living life like an open book—any page can be read by anyone—no secrets—no hiding.

Self-love is

- Discovering the greatness deep within me.
- Believing in my own preciousness and uniqueness.
- Knowing I am a beloved child of God.
- Knowing that within me resides the Spirit of God.
- Knowing I am a spiritual being having a human experience.
- Knowing I am Divine Faith
    Divine Strength
    Divine Love
    Divine Wisdom

Divine Power
Divine Will
Divine Understanding
Divine Imagination
Divine Zeal
Divine Order
Divine Renunciation/Elimination

Self-love is Experiencing God at work
o In me
o Through me
o Around me
- Being an open channel for the healing energy of love.
- Being God's love in action.

Self-love comes through
- Self-discovery
- Self-discipline
- Self-forgiveness
- Self-acceptance

Self-love produces
- Self-reliance
- Self-confidence
- An inner security
- An inner calm and peace
- Enthusiasm
- Health
- Harmony
- Success
- Happiness

## Steps to a Strong Self-Love

1. Get rid of your fears and your ego by processing them through the Twelve Steps.

2. Let your identity come forth and alive:
   A. Discover yourself with the Twelve Steps.
   B. Reveal yourself through the Twelve Steps.
   C. Be yourself: activate your twelve powers—practice your twelve life strengths.

3. Be good to yourself: Nurture yourself.
   Compliment yourself.
   Set new, safe boundaries.

4. Have compassion for yourself—forgive yourself.

5. Improve yourself: Keep on growing—be teachable.

   Allow feedback and mirroring by others.

6. Accept yourself: Be grateful for who you are.

7. Commit yourself to a great cause: Allow yourself to feel useful and to make a difference.

8. Believe in success: You are worthy of it. You are a precious child of God.

9. Strive for excellence: Do not settle for addictive patterns nor comfort zones. Give it your best!

10. Build self-love in others: Be involved in your support groups.
    Give unconditionally.
    Bless others and the blessing will return multiplied.

## A Love Story from a Wife in Recovery

When I was small, Mother packed the car for a visit to Grandmother. Then we drove to my dad's office to pick him up and begin our drive. But there was a long delay once we got to Dad's office. Mother parked the car, and we waited...and waited... and waited. With a child's impatience, I demanded to know where Daddy was. Mother answered, "Oh, he probably just got tied up."

It was the first time I had heard this expression, and I was shocked. *who tied my daddy up?!* I demanded, alarmed that he needed our help and irritated that Mother was so nonchalant about it.

This childhood incident is a very good illustration of my relationship with my parents. My father was the first alcoholic I loved. I experienced his anger and self-loathing, but I could also see his great heart and his innate goodness. I felt that, in ways I didn't understand, my daddy was "tied up," and I wanted desperately to set him free.

Mother, on the other hand, seemed nonchalant. I used to beg her to leave him, but she always said, "Your father is a good provider." Not college educated and with a history of ill health, Mother felt unprepared to go out into the world on her own—or maybe it was just easier to stay—or maybe she didn't believe in divorce. I don't know what held her there so long.

"Your father is a good provider" is the only compliment I remember Mother giving Dad. Other comments about him were critical and judgmental. In those days, people didn't understand alcoholism; they thought it was a sin—moral depravity. This was especially true of Mother, who had been raised by "hard-shell Baptist" parents. So Mother lived from a self-righteous perspective. She used to tell me, "Get a good education. Never have to depend on a man."

I was the oldest, so as soon as I got out of college, I married into a family of nondrinkers and moved to another state. I truly believed I had escaped any ill effects from my upbringing. Dad continued to drink, and my younger brother and sister experienced more severe consequences of his alcoholism as his disease progressed.

Finally, Mother heard about Al-Anon and began to attend. Within a few years, Dad bottomed out, and she left him. But I knew Dad needed help, and I made the arrangements for him to be admitted to a treatment center. He completed the treatment; we all received letters making amends, and things seemed to be getting better.

But AA didn't "take" for Dad. He attended only the minimum number of meetings the treatment center had recommended and then dropped out. Mother decided that if he wasn't going to AA, she wasn't going to Al-Anon, and they entered a period that stretched into years of a dry drunk/untreated Al-Anon relationship until finally, after forty-three years of marriage, Dad filed for divorce. He quickly married his widowed high school sweetheart, who hadn't been around for the tough years and didn't realize how precious and hard-earned sobriety was for him. Without any support, he began drinking again and died sooner than I was ready to let him go.

As for Mom, all those years of squelching her anger and putting up with unacceptable behavior took its toll on her. The divorce infuriated her, and her anger rolled out in great waves—an anger that went with her into the grave. As far as I could tell, neither of them ever forgave the other.

Meanwhile, after twenty-five years of marriage, I divorced my first husband and three years later, married the love of my life—my soul mate. He was fun and gregarious.

On our fourth anniversary, I woke up to my worst nightmare, married to an alcoholic. I was horrified because I had promised myself as a little girl that no man would ever treat me the way Dad treated Mother. But my beloved husband had done that very thing, and I knew I had to take action and keep my promise to myself.

So I clearly remember that morning as I contemplated my situation. As I sat in bed in the early morning, something within me said, "It's time for you to make friends with this disease." From Mother's experience, I knew what to do. Immediately, I started going to Al-Anon and have continued ever since.

I waited for the effects of my husband's binge to wear off. (I had learned from Dad that it's pointless to talk to an alcoholic while he's drunk.) Then I confronted him with my observation that he might be an alcoholic.

His response was, "You're right. I do drink too much. I'll stop. Okay?" I thank God for my experience with Dad because I knew this would not be enough. I knew what a dry drunk is like. So I said, "No. That won't be enough."

To which he responded, "Well, I won't go to counseling. I will not go to treatment. And I sure as hell won't work a Ten-Step program."

When I heard this, something within me giggled, although my outward demeanor was very serious, and this giggle said, "He's just going to die when he finds out there are twelve."

Clearly, this journey was not going to be easy. I got help, not only from Al-Anon but also from trusted counselors. I waited several days until my head got clear and I knew what I must do.

I love my husband. The thought of leaving him broke my heart. But I knew what I was up against, and I had made myself a promise that I intended to keep. So, when I was ready, I handed him a packet of information about a treatment center and asked him to go. He was furious. He took that packet and threw it across the room. "No" was his answer.

I was prepared. I said, "I'll give you ten days to think about it. I'm going out of town. If you still feel this way when I get back, I will immediately file for divorce." And I walked out.

It was the hardest thing I've ever done.

I felt defeated and afraid. *Powerless.*

Just as the Twelve Steps promise, a Higher Power took over and did for me what I could not do for myself. Many unexplained coincidences occurred—I call them miracles. People with the information I needed at that moment appeared. And I intuitively knew what to do next. I took one step at a time—one day at a time.

My husband and I were separated for eight months, during which I worked with a sponsor and went to as many as three Al-Anon meetings some days. We were also working with a marriage counselor. My husband wanted to reconcile, but I wasn't at all sure that was what I wanted. I needed more time.

During this period of separation, I learned to love myself. I began to heal. I yielded to my emotions and told him how I truly felt, without judging myself as to whether my feelings were "nice" or "acceptable." Each time I got clear on an action I needed to take, I did it. I didn't care whether anyone else liked it or not. I was being true to myself.

But for months, I was not able to forgive my husband. The breakthrough finally came on a day after I had attended a noon Al-Anon meeting. It was my turn to see our marriage counselor by myself, and as I seated myself on the couch, I dissolved into tears. I said, "I know I should forgive him, but I can't." The counselor let me sit there and cry until I was finished.

When I looked up, my resentment for my husband's actions had vanished, and it has never returned. In fact, right now, I can't remember exactly what I was so upset about. This was a dramatic experience of God doing for me what I was not able to do. I had surrendered, and forgiveness came.

Within the year, my husband had done everything he said he would not do—AA, counseling, and treatment. When I went for family week to the treatment center, I found a husband who was at peace with himself. He asked me to go through the same treatment he had received. Fortunately, this treatment center used the Desjardins model. It didn't limit its services to alcoholics; I qualified as a codependent and workaholic, and the treatment I received there is one of the greatest blessings of my life.

For the last nine years, we have been a couple in recovery. We have sponsors. We attend AA and Al-Anon meetings. We work the program.

It hasn't been easy. About four years into recovery, we found ourselves on the brink of divorce again. But this time, instead of telling him what he had to do, I started praying for him. I was so furious that I couldn't bring myself to ask God to give him good things, but I could ask that God be with him, so that's what I did. After a week or two of great distress, we were able to reconcile. A few days afterward, I found the courage to ask him what did it. What had convinced him to stay and try again? His answer was, "I talked to my sponsor, and he suggested I pray for you. So that's what I've been doing." So—I was praying for him, he was praying for me, and God was again doing the work of forgiveness and reconciliation.

I work a good Al-Anon program, but sometimes even that isn't enough to meet the challenges of being in a recovery marriage. Recently, I had another meltdown when my husband attacked me verbally, and I became so angry I could not get over it. I felt this should not be happening after almost nine years in recovery.

Fortunately, Gilles and Liliane Desjardins live nearby, and I knew of their transformative work through a four-day process called the Inner Journey. I called Liliane and was able to get into her next session. This work begins with discovering imprints—patterns learned in childhood that drive our behavior.

The "AHA!" for me during this session was twofold:

I was untrusting.

Like a silent, invisible ticker tape, my mother's old messages were unconsciously running through my brain. I was accepting unacceptable behavior, numbing out emotionally, and not respecting my husband by telling him the truth about the effect of his words and actions on me. The ticker tape of criticism was drowning out the truth.

These realizations have brought me into more complete truthfulness. Therefore, I am at greater peace. I've made a new commitment not to run away emotionally when his behavior gets difficult, but to stay engaged, asking God to do for me what I cannot do.

Like my father, my husband has a great heart. He's a good man, and I love him. I'm learning to love him better, and today I have great compassion for him and the challenge of his journey. I also have compassion for myself.

"And practice these principles in all our affairs" are the last words of the Twelve Steps. Those principles are humility, honesty, hope, love, and purity of intent.

Today, I'm focused on practicing those principles in my marriage, as well as in every area of my life.

Today, I feel blessed to be married to an alcoholic in recovery. I feel it is my life's purpose to be happily married to him. We are helping each other heal.

In the earliest days of this journey, someone told me there wasn't much hope for my husband's recovery. I took this information to my trusted counselor, who said, "That isn't true! Recovery is possible. Look at Gerald and Betty Ford. They created a beautiful love story."

At that moment, I decided that was what I wanted—a beautiful love story. In God's grace, that story is still unfolding.

"Within an instant, love can transform the world."
Author Unknown

# Bibliography

A.A. Services. (1976) *Alcoholics Anonymous: Big Book.* (3rd Ed.) Alcoholics Anonymous World Services, Inc.

Beattie, M. (1990) *The language of letting go.* Hazelden Foundation.

Beiler, J. and Smucker, S. (2009) *thinks no evil: The inside story of the amish schoolhouse shooting...and beyond.* Howard Books.

Berk, P.M. (2006) *Mountain's stillness river's wisdom: A compassionate guide to the art of being.* Booksurge.

Conyers, B. (2003) *Addict in the family: stories of loss, hope, and recovery.* Hazelden Foundation.

Coombs, R.H., Ed. (2004) *Handbook of addictive disorders: a practical guide to diagnosis and treatment.* John Wiley & Sons.

*Courage to Change.* (1992) Al-Anon Family Group Headquarters.

Frederiksen, L. (2008) *If You Loved Me, You'd Stop!* KLJ Publishing.

*From Survival to Recovery.* (2000) Al-Anon Family Group Headquarters.

Gorski, Terence and Merlene Miller. (1986) *Staying Sober: A Guide for Relapse Prevention.* Independence Press.

Hawkins, D.R. (2002) *Power vs. Force: The Hidden Determinants of Human Behavior.* Hay House.

*How Al-Anon Works for Families and Friends of Alcoholics.* (1995) Al-Anon Family Group Headquarters, Inc.

Judith, A. (2006) *Waking the Global Heart.* Elite Books.

LeDoux, Joseph. (1996) *The Emotional Brain: The Mysterious Underpinnings of Emotional Life.* Simon and Schuster.

Moyers, William Cope. (2006) *Broken.* Penguin Books.

Oelklaus, Nancy. (2008) *Journey from Head to Heart: Living and Working Authentically.* Loving Healing Press.

Ryan, Christa Jan. (2008) *Silent Screams from the Hamptons.* Robert Reed Publishers.

Satir, Virginia. (1990) *Peoplemaking*. Condor Books.

Sinor, Barbara. (2009) *Addiction: what's really going on? Inside a heroin treatment program* . Ann Arbor: Loving Healing Press.

Sinor, Barbara. (2003) *An inspirational guide for the recovering soul*. Astra.

The Al-Anon Family Groups: Classic Edition. (2000) Al-Anon Family Group Headquarters.

Watson, Irene. (2009) *The sitting swing: Finding wisdom to know the difference*. Loving Healing Press.

Wegscheider-Cruse, Sharon. (1989) *Another chance: hope and health for the alcoholic family*. Science and Behavior Books.

Wegscheider-Cruse, Sharon. (1996) *Family Reconstruction: The Living Theater Model*. Science and Behavior Books.

# Appendix: Additional Resources

Austin Recovery
8402 Cross Park Drive
Austin, TX 78754
800.373.2081
**www.austinrecovery.org**

Head to Heart
5400 Mt. Bonnell Road
Austin, TX 78731
512. 431.4946
**www.headtoheart.com**

Higher Power Productions
115 Golf Crest Cove
Lakeway, TX 78734
877. 477.5483
**www.higherpower.info**

## Website Resources

Al-Anon/Alateen
 **www.al-anon.org**

Co-Anon Family Groups
**www.co-anon.org**

Codependents Anonymous
**www.coda.org**

Rewriting Life Scripts
**www.rewritinglifescripts.com**

# About the Authors

**Liliane Desjardins** was born in Zagreb, Croatia and educated in Paris, France. Her background is liturgical arts and one of her outstanding works are the stained glass windows at the Catholic Chapel at Kennedy International Airport, New York. Upon entering recovery from addictions Liliane's focus shifted from aesthetic beauty to reshaping and re-creating her life and the lives of others.

Liliane is a Certified Clinical Addiction Specialist. She is renowned for her highly successful and innovative work and the Desjardins Unified Model of Treatment of Addictions. She is the co-founder of Pavilion Gilles Desjardins in Val David, Quebec, Canada and Pavillon International a center for treatment of addictions in NC. She has 32 years of experience in clinical work.

Liliane has a profound and passionate dedication to her work, which is rooted in 35 years of personal recovery. Liliane is a proven leader in the healing of emotions and deep seated self-defeating belief systems and addictions. She has brought hope and healing to thousands.

After retiring from Pavillon, Liliane and her husband Gilles moved to Austin, Texas. Liliane is president of Higher Power Productions. Her focus is now on empowering individuals to access their Authentic Self and actualize their potential. She enjoys playing golf with her husband Gilles and playing with their adorable little dog named Angel.

**Nancy Oelklaus** lives on the rim of a canyon in Austin, Texas, with her husband, Harlan, and Feathers, a curly white lap dog. Nancy lightens the load for leaders and ordinary people by teaching them powerful findings from neuroscience ignited by the scriptural wisdom of the ages. Her professional and personal clients learn to create environments where people thrive, at work and at home. Specializing in helping people make transitions, her knowledge and skills have been learned through more than 30 years of working in education and business to understand how adults learn and change—and how they can do it faster so that they may spend more time in "happily ever-after."

Dr. Oelklaus holds a BA in communications/theater education from Oklahoma Baptist University, an MA in English from the University of North Texas, and a doctorate in educational administration from Texas A&M University in Commerce. She is the author of

*Journey From Head to Heart: Living and Working Authentically*, and *Alphabet Meditations for Teachers: Everyday Wisdom for Educator*s. Nancy enjoys taking photographs and writing poetry.

**Irene Watson** holds a Masters Degree in Psychology, with honors, from Regis University in Denver, CO. Her emphasis was spirituality and psychosynthesis. Irene's life has taken her on many paths, with breakthrough results and exemplar growth, to find her authentic and true self. She has designed and facilitated workshops and retreats in the United States and Canada. At present she is the Managing Editor of her book review and author publicity company, Reader Views. Irene is the author of *The Sitting Swing: Finding Wisdom to Know the Difference, Authors Access: 30 Success Secrets for Authors and Publishers*, and editor of *The Story That Must Be Told: True Tales of Transformation*. She lives with her husband on the banks of Barton Creek in Austin, Texas along with their Pomeranian, Tafton, a rescued cat, Patches, and rescued cockatiels, Clement and Elgin.

# Index

# How You Can Help Support the Higher Power Foundation

*Rewriting Life Scripts: Transformational Recovery for Families of Addicts* has been published in conjunction with Higher Power Foundation Inc. as a fundraiser as well as providing this book free of charge to families when a family member undergoes treatment. All proceeds go directly to support the means. The authors have not and will not take compensation or any of the proceeds.

Higher Power Foundation Inc. was established to provide financial support to individuals needing assistance in attending spiritual based workshops, retreats, and programs. It operates within the meaning of Section 501(c)(3) of the Internal Revenue Code of 1954. Any donations are tax-deductable.

Your involvement is accepted by:

1. Making a direct contribution to Higher Power Foundation to be used for scholarships.

2. Making a contribution allotted to providing books to families of addicts returning from treatment at no charge.

3. Making a contribution allotted to providing books to a specific center or group.

4. Becoming a sponsor for a minimum of 3000 books. A full page sponsorship acknowledgment will be placed in the books.

For more information on how you can get involved please contact:
www.HigherPowerFoundation.com
info@higherpowerfoundation.com

Breinigsville, PA USA
29 March 2010
235172BV00002B/2/P

9 781932 690972